A.J.MASON.

ORTHOPTIC ASSESSMENT
AND MANAGEMENT

Modern Optometry

SERIES EDITOR

R. FLETCHER

MScTech, FBOA, HD, FSMC (Hons),
D'Orth, DCLP
Emeritus Professor, City University, London
Docent II, Kongsberg Inginør Hogskøle,
Kongsberg, Norge

OTHER BOOKS IN THE SERIES

Glaucoma in Optometric Practice
F.G. BROWN and R. FLETCHER

Eye Examination and Refraction
R.J. ALLEN, R. FLETCHER
and D.C. STILL

*Optometric Management of
Visual Handicap*
HELEN FARRALL

Orthoptic Assessment and Management

DAVID STIDWILL

FBCO, DCLP

Optometrist, Visiting Clinician, Aston University
Honorary Secretary, Orthoptic and Binocular Vision Association
Member of Assessment Board, The British College of Optometrists

MODERN OPTOMETRY

OXFORD

BLACKWELL SCIENTIFIC PUBLICATIONS

LONDON EDINBURGH

BOSTON MELBOURNE PARIS BERLIN VIENNA

© 1990 by David Stidwill

Blackwell Scientific Publications
Editorial offices:
Osney Mead, Oxford OX2 0EL
25 John Street, London WC1N 2BL
23 Ainslie Place, Edinburgh EH3 6AJ
3 Cambridge Center, Suite 208
   Cambridge, Massachusetts 02142, USA
54 University Street, Carlton
   Victoria 3053, Australia

First published 1990

Set by Setrite Typesetters Ltd
Printed and bound in Great Britain by
the University Press, Cambridge

DISTRIBUTORS

Marston Book Services Ltd
PO Box 87
Oxford OX2 0DT
(*Orders*: Tel: 0865 791155
         Fax: 0865 791927
         Telex: 837515

USA
   Mosby-Year Book, Inc.
   200 North LaSalle Street
   Chicago, Illinois 60601
   (*Orders*: Tel: (312) 726−9733)

Canada
   Mosby-Year Book, Inc.
   5240 Finch Avenue East
   Scarborough, Ontario
   (*Orders*: Tel: (416) 298−1588)

Australia
   Blackwell Scientific Publications
      (Australia) Pty Ltd
   54 University Street
   Carlton, Victoria 3053
   (*Orders*: Tel: (03) 347−0300)

British Library
Cataloguing in Publication Data

Stidwill, David
   Orthoptic assessment and management.
   1. Orthoptics
   I. Title
   617.762
ISBN 0−632−02776−2

Contents

Preface

This is one book in a series covering the syllabus of the professional qualifying examination of the British College of Optometrists. The aim has been to produce a text which bridges the differences between general ophthalmic services, and community and hospital orthoptic practice. In addition to the pre-registration optometrist, the approach should appeal to the established practitioner and orthoptist. References to recent papers and leading texts are included.

The first chapters cover the growth of normal visual functions, and failures of their development. The clinical investigation of patients follows, together with the classification and management of motor and sensory anomalies. The final chapters are on neurological anomalies of binocular vision, and examination preparation. The appendices give case histories, revision questions and a glossary.

With the advent of shared information, patient management in the future should be a team effort where health professionals can communicate effectively. It is hoped that this book will provide a further step in that direction.

David Stidwill

Acknowledgements

I would like to thank Mr R. Ackerley, MSc, FBOA, FSMC and Mrs A. Bishop, BSc, FBCO, DBO for their comments on the text; Mrs J. Pearsall and Miss S. Higgs for word processing; Messrs Clement Clarke International, Harlow, for Figures 4.1 to 4.4, 5.6, 5.7, 6.7, and for Hess screen charts; Andrew and Peter Stidwill for word processing and Figures 6.5 to 6.11. The line illustrations were drawn by Mrs C. Taylor. I must thank some anonymous patients for agreeing to allow inclusion of photographs and Hess plots. I am indebted to the authors of the texts and papers which I have cited. Finally I must thank Professor R. Fletcher for advice in every aspect of preparing the text and figures, and also Mr R. Miles of Blackwell Scientific Publications Ltd.

Abbreviations

The following abbreviations are in clinical use and are used in this text. In American use the 'O' is deleted, e.g. XT instead of XOT.

XOT: exotropia
XOP: exophoria
XOP/T: intermittent exotropia
SOT: esotropia
SOP: esophoria
SOP/T: intermittent esotropia
HP: hyperphoria

Hypertropia and hypotropia: not abbreviated. The abbreviations R/L and L/R are deprecated since they do not indicate whether a phoria or a tropia is being described, and if a tropia, which eye is fixing.

R: right
L: left
A: alternating
DVD: dissociated vertical deviation
RMR: right medial rectus
RLR, RSR, RIR, RIO, RSO: the other extra-ocular muscles of the right eye
NPC: near point of convergence
NRC: normal retinal correspondence
ARC: anomalous retinal correspondence
HARC, UHARC: harmonious, unharmonious ARC
BSV: binocular single vision
V: vision (unaided)
VA: visual acuity (with a refractive correction)
DS: dioptre sphere
DC: dioptre cylinder
Δ.   prism dioptre

VER, VECP:	visual evoked response, visual evoked cortical potentials
AC/A:	accommodative convergence/accommodation ratio (in prism dioptres/dioptres of accommodation)
MLF:	medial longitudinal fasciculus
PPRF:	paramedian pontine reticular formation
P.Q.E.:	the professional qualifying examination of the British College of Optometrists

CHAPTER 1
Normal and Abnormal Binocular Vision

1.1 Development of normal binocular vision

At birth the eye is about one-third of the adult size. The cornea is nearly adult size. The histological development of the fovea is not complete until 6 months old. Visual acuity obtained by optokinetic nystagmus and preferential looking techniques is around 6/330 (Thompson and Drasdo, 1988), see Table 1.1. Conjugate fixation and following may be seen from birth but certainly from 4 to 6 weeks of age. Roving conjugate eye movements change to deliberate following when the child is presented with a large moving object such as a face. Visual attention can be detected in a newborn baby by the reduction of other motor

Table 1.1 Development of visual acuity (measured by preferential looking: Teller Acuity Cards) (Gwiazda *et al.*, 1980; McDonald *et al.*, 1986).

Age	Binocular Acuity	Monocular Acuity
Newborn	6/120−6/360	No data
1 month	6/90−6/360	6/120−6/480
2 months	6/36−6/180	6/60−6/240
4 months	6/24−6/90	6/30−6/120
6 months	6/15−6/90	6/24−6/90
9 months	6/15−6/90	6/24−6/90
12 months	6/15−6/90	6/24−6/90
18 months	6/12−6/30	6/15−6/45
24 months	6/9−6/24	6/12−6/30
30 months	6/6−6/15	6/6−6/15
36 months	6/5−6/12	6/5−6/12

Other measurements of acuity at birth are as follows: Brown and Yamamoto, (1986), 0.69 cycles/degree (binocular); Dobson *et al.*, (1987), 1.00 cycles/degree (binocular); Thompson and Drasdo, (1988), 0.64 cycles/degree (binocular); Thompson and Drasdo (1988), 0.55 cycles/degree (monocular).

activity, widening of the palpebral apertures and slow regular breathing. However, hunger, pain or sleepiness following a feed will reduce the baby's attention.

Brief independent eye movements may occur in the first 6 months but a persistent convergent or divergent position of one eye is abnormal. During this period some degree of intermittent exotropia is frequently seen (Sondhi *et al.*, 1988). This awaits further confirmation. Esotropia in the first 6 months may affect 0.1% of all babies (derived from Adelstein *et al.*, 1967, and von Noorden, 1985).

Optokinetic nystagmus (fixation and following response) is reflexly present in the neonate independently of the baby's state of attention. It is evidence of the absence of blindness. However, blind children will make a 'dolls eye movement'. When the head is passively turned in one direction, the eyes move together in the opposite direction. The horizontal response is present at birth and the vertical response by 2 months. This response depends upon the non-optic reflexes stimulated by the vestibular system and the proprioceptive neck reflex. It can be used to test motility and vestibular function, although in normal children the fixation reflex tends to override the doll's eye movement after the age of 3 months.

The direct and consensual light reflexes appear 30 weeks post-conception; from this time the head is jerked back in a protective reaction when a bright light is shone on a premature baby (Peiper's reflex). Blinking to light occurs even in sleep, but to a threatening hand movement, not until the eighth week of life. Lid movements may not be conjugate during the first 2 months.

Preferential looking visual acuities are often measured in cycles per degree (c/°), which describes the width of the square wave targets used in this technique. As a rough guide, infant acuity in cycles per degree equals the age in months. The versions of these tests which are (or will be) available as cards for routine visual acuity testing of children from birth up to the age of 3 to 5 years old, include the Teller Acuity Cards, the Keeler Acuity Cards (designed by A.Fielder, Professor of Ophthalmology at Birmingham University, UK), and the proposed Mallett preferential looking test.

Cycloplegic refraction at birth averages +2.00 DS and decreases to +0.50 DS by 5 years. Average anisometropia is just under 0.50 DS at birth and about

Table 1.2 Conversion: Cycles/degree to Snellen acuity.

10 c/°	= 6/18
7.5 c/°	= 6/24
5.0 c/°	= 6/36
3.0 c/°	= 6/60
1.5 c/°	= 6/120 (3/60)
0.75 c/°	= 6/240
0.5 c/°	= 6/360 (1/60)

0.10 DS by 1 year (Thompson and Drasdo, 1988). Similarly, bilateral astigmatism of around 1.50 dioptres in the neonate reduces to 0.50 dioptres by 18 months (Mohindra *et al.*, 1978; Atkinson *et al.*, 1980). In the author's experience, astigmatism of that degree is found in 50% of babies who are selected only on the grounds that there is a family history of (any) refractive error. Accommodation is slow to adjust during the first 2 months and a non-cycloplegic refraction may well show an apparent myopia of −4.00 DS. By 6 months accommodation is fully active and accommodative strabismus is increasingly possible. Convergence is evident by 3 months. There is evidence that the higher neural centres start to process retinal disparity information to produce stereopsis from 4 months and clinically the Lang random dot stereopsis test will produce a positive response (a change of fixation from target to target) from 6 months in a significant proportion of infants. Conversely, difficulty in fusing the images from each eye in an infant with squint or anisometropia, is likely to cause the development of suppression from this age.

The fixation disparity reflex can be tested from 6 to 8 months using a 10^Δ test. This is based on the classic 4^Δ test, (see 5.14). By 9 months the more sophisticated Lang test will produce a grasp reflex onto its stereoscopic targets. The fixation disparity reflex and fusional amplitudes continue to develop and to become more robust up to the age of 8 years. A fusional response has been shown experimentally in neonates (Friedrich and de Decker, 1987).

1.2   Clinical aspects of visual development

In the management of anomalies of binocular vision there are three critical ages for decisions about treatment to be taken: 12 weeks, 24 months and 8 years. Operation for congenital monocular cataracts gives a better prognosis if performed before 12 weeks. This is the *critical period for fixation*. Early onset squint has a better binocular function if surgery is completed before the first 24 months. This is the *critical period for acuity*. It is equivalent to the 'critical period' in experimental animals, (see Blakemore, 1974, and for humans, based on the effect of meridional amblyopia, Mitchell *et al.*, 1973). Thirdly, there is a *plastic period* where the fixation reflex and vergence control can be lost, up to the age of approximately 8 years. During this period the peak onset of squint occurs, between 2 and 3 years old, due to the increasing visual demands made by a longer active day. From 8 years old the response to a sudden change in motor or sensory input may be diplopia rather than adaptations such as suppression, anomalous correspondence or eccentric fixation. For example, after 8 years old either a traumatic squint or surgery for a long-standing squint may each produce diplopia. More rarely, excessive amblyopia treatment can also produce diplopia when carried out after this age, where it also produces a change in the squint angle, particularly in deep ARC. However, a gradual change in motor or sensory status may still produce suppression − the first stage in sensory adaptation.

Equally, judicious amblyopia treatment and squint surgery can be safely under-taken in teenagers and adults.

Experimental work showing a loss in binocularly driven cortical cells has been thought to contra-indicate vigorous occlusion therapy. However, it appears that it is the experimentally-induced strabismus which produces the loss rather than occlusion. Consequently occlusion is still used as the main treatment of amblyopia, although with safeguards to avoid stimulus deprivation amblyopia of the occluded eye (von Noorden, 1985).

1.3   Development of abnormal binocular vision

The reader should refer to a textbook of paediatric ophthalmology for a discussion of general ocular developmental abnormalities, (see Helveston and Ellis, 1983). Table 1.3 lists some syndromes which include strabismus.

Table 1.3 Strabismus related syndromes.

Disorder	Characteristics
Apert's syndrome	Nystagmus, exophthalmos, keratopathy, optic atrophy
Benedikt's syndrome	Red nucleus lesion, ipsilateral III nerve paresis, contralateral half-body paresis
Cri du chat syndrome	Hypertelorism, decreased lacrimation, retinal vessel tortuosity
Crouzon's disease (craniofacial dystosis)	Nystagmus, exophthalmos, decreased vision, anterior facial asymmetry
Down's syndrome (trisomy 21)	Epicanthal folds, oblique palebral fissures, muscular hypotony
Ehlers-Danlos disease	Ptosis, extra-ocular muscle hypotony, hyper-elastic skin, keratoconus, lens subluxation, retinopathy
Hurler's disease (mucopolysaccharidosis)	Ptosis, keratopathy, optic atrophy
Laurence-Moon-Biedl-Bardet syndrome	Nystagmus, ophthalmoplegia, optic atrophy, polydactyly
Marfan's syndrome	Nystagmus, lens subluxation, arachnodactyly, heart defect
Millard-Gubler syndrome	VI nerve paresis, hemiplegia of leg and arm
Parry-Romberg disease	Horner's syndrome, enophthalmos, progressive facial hemiatrophy
Pierre-Robin syndrome	Possible high myopia, cleft palate, respiratory distress, micrognathia
Rubella (congenital)	Microphthalmos, glaucoma, cataract, deafness, heart disease, mental retardation
Turner's syndrome	Epicanthal folds, neck webbing, low set ears, gonadal dysgenesis

Early onset concomitant squint includes:

1 Infantile esotropia (synonyms: congenital squint, cross-fixation esotropia) which develops in the first 6 months with the right eye used for left gaze and vice versa sometimes with an accompanying head turn towards the side being fixated. Bilateral weakness of the lateral recti muscles is possibly due to delayed development. The eventual outcome as an alternating or unilateral squint, or non-accommodative esophoria depends upon the speed of development. There may also be dissociated vertical deviation and latent or manifest nystagmus.

2 Early onset accommodative esotropia presenting before six months of age with associated hypermetropia and often a high AC/A ratio.

3 Nystagmus blockage esotropia (synonym: nystagmus blockage syndrome) where congenital horizontal nystagmus increases in amplitude when the deviated eye straightens.

4 Early onset exotropia. Recent work has shown a significant number of intermittent exotropias occurring up to 6 months. The minority which persist may show dissociated vertical deviation and possibly nystagmus.

5 Post-paretic esotropia. Transient sixth nerve paresis may leave an esotropia which becomes concomitant − but look for a slight lateral rectus underaction, or a medial rectus overaction. A transient sixth nerve paresis may be caused by birth trauma. During the first 2 years, viral infections causing pyrexia or upper respiratory infection can also cause a transient sixth nerve paresis which may completely disappear after a few weeks or months but leave a post-paretic esotropia. There may be a constant head turn. Nystagmus and dissociated vertical deviation are not present.

6 Heterotropia associated with congenital pareses. *Congenital pareses* include:
 (i) Duane's syndrome which, though not inherited, is associated with other neural and skeletal abnormalities and often produces concomitant squint in the next generation.
 (ii) Benedikt's syndrome: unilateral third nerve paresis.
 (iii) Brown's syndrome: fusion of the superior oblique tendon sheath with the trochlea (simulating an inferior oblique paresis), (see 8.12).
 (iv) Congenital abducens paresis.
 (v) Horizontal strabismus fixus: bilateral esotropia.
 (vi) Moebius' syndrome: paresis of sixth and seventh cranial nerves.

From 6 months a *partially accommodative squint* (first type) may appear showing both hypermetropia and anomalies of muscle insertions. Other anomalies include hypoplasia or absence of the muscles, and abnormal check ligaments (or other fibrous bands connecting the muscles and the orbital walls). More typically the onset is between 1 and 3 years. A *fully accommodative squint* may also appear in the first year of life though more commonly between 2 and 5 years. If a fully accommodative squint is neglected, a partially accommodative squint (second type) may develop due to sensory and motor adaptations to the deviation. These include medial rectus hypertrophy (von Noorden, 1985).

Exotropia is usually intermittent in early childhood but may become constant spontaneously or associated with myopia in teenagers, or with reduction of accommodation in adults.

Amblyopia due to stimulus deprivation – e.g. congenital cataract or secondary to anisometropia, high bilateral ametropia, or strabismus may occur during the first months of life or at any age up to 8 years. A traumatic cataract after that age would reduce VA, but would decreasingly cause actual amblyopia. Conversely the treatment of amblyopia will be much slower after 8 years of age.

Decompensation of heterophoria may occur whenever additional stresses are placed on the vergence eye movement system.

Decompensation of a congenital paresis may occur when stress or ill health break down the adaption to the paresis. In other words, a paretic heterophoria becomes decompensated and is then an intermittent or constant paretic squint. Intermittent diplopia may occur when the patient is tired, though typically with less disturbance than in an acquired paresis.

Convergence insufficiency can occur suddenly in schoolchildren and the diplopia and disorientation may alarm child, parent and practitioner. In teenagers the onset may be associated with examination stress or a first job. Accommodative insufficiency occurs in about a quarter of convergence insufficiency patients but can occur independently. It may be associated with ill health, e.g. glandular fever, head trauma, some types of therapeutic and non-therapeutic drugs including ethanol.

In early adulthood, undercorrected hypermetropia in esotropia may produce intermittent diplopia as a greater accommodative effort is needed to see clearly. Early presbyopia may produce a variety of symptoms, for example accommodative lag on looking from near vision to distance vision may be associated with a decompensated exophoria. Compensating the deviation may reduce the synergistic use of accommodation and convergence to control the exophoria. A fixation disparity test may show under, over or full compensation in such circumstances.

Age related exotropia occurs independently of vision reduction and may be preceded by a decompensated exophoria. Age related eye movement anomalies may produce diplopia on looking to left or right and reduced pursuit or fixation control.

1.4   Prevalence and differential diagnosis of squint

The general prevalence of strabismus is around 2.5% (von Noorden, (1985) and Scheie and Albert, (1977) – 2.0%; Frandsen, (1960) – 5%), of which 10% is

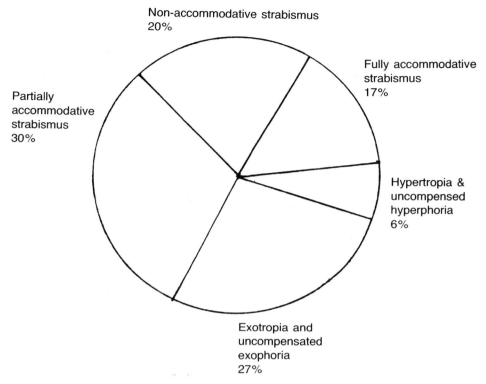

Fig. 1.1 The incidence of deviation categories in 1760 ophthalmic patients with strabismus or uncompensated heterophoria. (D.B. Stidwill: previously unpublished data.)

fully accommodative, 35% partially accommodative and 25% non-accommodative (and see Fig. 1.1).

The prevalence of strabismus in the following categories is:

Negroes (USA)	0.1% squint
Premature babies	18% squint
Birth trauma	45% squint
Down's syndrome	50% squint
Brain damage	53% squint

If a parent squints the risk to their children is ten times greater, i.e 25% squint. If there is a family history of strabismus and the child has a refractive error of +2.00 DS or more, the incidence of squint is 86%. Over +3.50 DS in the more hypermetropic meridian by the age of 1 year carries a 45% risk of amblyopia and squint (Ingram, 1986). Its correction in infancy drops the incidence to normal levels (Atkinson *et al.*, 1987).

Congenital cataract will cause amblyopia and possibly strabismus. The incidence is 1 in 10 000 live births: 25% of all neonatal blind registrations are due to cataract. Causes include rubella, use of steroids by the mother, or Still's disease causing uveitis and secondary cataract. There is also a large number of syndromes involving cataract. A squint is the presenting feature in 20% of retinoblastomas which have an incidence of 1 in 18 000 with an average onset age of 12 months.

Retinopathy of prematurity associated with a birth weight of 500 g or less, or with excess oxygen, causes peripheral cicatrization in 20% of cases, with disc dragging and strabismus in some children due to the ectopic macula.

Strabismus may be seen in non-accidental injury to children, who may appear abnormally sullen or avoid eye contact. In these cases retinal haemorrhages may also be present.

The age distribution of squint onset is 15% (0−1 years), 21% (1−2 years), 25% (2−3 years), 18% (3−4 years), 10% (4−5 years) and 1% (5 years), (Adelstein and Scully, 1967). The median age of squint onset is 21 months (non-accommodative), 30 months (partially accommodative), and 30 months (fully accommodative), (Graham, 1974). Convergence insufficiency (>12 cm) affects 5% of schoolchildren (Ackerley, unpublished data).

1.5   Pseudo-strabismus

Pseudo-strabismus (synonym: pseudo-tropia) is an appearance of squint when the visual axes are not deviated. Pseudo-tropia may co-exist with an intermittent heterotropia. It should not be dismissed without a full assessment, and a later review.

Pseudo-esotropia

This may be caused by:

1 Epicanthal folds due to the low bridge of the nose in normal infants. Epicanthal folds can persist as a congenital familial anomaly.
2 Facial asymmetry: in telecanthus the orbits are normal, but the medial canthi are abnormally separated due to soft tissue hypertrophy. Facial asymmetry can also occur in cranial dysgenesis such as Crouzon's disease, and other syndromes such as Turner's syndrome (see Table 1.3).
3 Negative angle lambda: the corneal light reflex is displaced temporally.
4 Hypotelorism: a narrow skull with a narrow interpupillary distance.

Pseudo-exotropia

This may be caused by:

1 Hypertelorism: a wide interpupillary distance.
2 Exophthalmos.
3 Ectopic macula: the macula of one eye is dragged temporally due to the contraction of choroid and retinal lesions in choroiditis or in retinopathy of prematurity.
4 Positive angle lambda: the corneal light reflex is displaced nasally.

Pseudo-hypertropia

Pseudo-hypertropia may be due to unilateral ptosis, unilateral coloboma, or where one eye is higher than the other, as a congenital or acquired anomaly. This latter should be distinguished from a 'skew gaze' deviation (see 9.11), in which bifoveal fixation is *not* present.

CHAPTER 2

Background: Orthoptic Terminology, Surgical Principles, the Development of Orthoptic Techniques

2.1   Orthoptic terminology

Orthoptics has suffered from a plethora of terminology which is slowly falling into order. Duane's classification of motor anomalies into defects of convergence and divergence, although useful, produces a confusion between static defects of ocular motor deviation and defects of the dynamic ability to converge and diverge. Some terminology may be considered of dubious value. For example the division of alternating heterotropia into 'essential' and 'accidental' depending on whether the condition is freely alternating, or with fixation preference for one eye. It is simpler to write 'AXOT' or 'RXOT (can alternate)'. The terms 'morphoscopic VA' for linear VA and 'angular VA' for single letter VA, though popular recently, have theoretical objections (see von Noorden, 1985).

Obsolete terminology is discussed at 4.9. The term 'paradoxical diplopia' should be called 'unharmonious ARC with diplopia'. It occurs briefly after surgery while the previous ARC has not yet been suppressed. The 'blind spot syndrome' where the fixation image falls on the blind spot of the deviated eye, is now felt to be a fortuitous rather than a deliberate response.

In Table 2.1, the most appropriate term is given first. The term 'deviation' is currently used as a generic description which includes both heterotropia and heterophoria. In the past this term was used to describe a supra-nuclear anomaly of gaze (see 9.11).

2.2   Surgical principles

When examining a patient, it is often possible to detect signs of previous strabismus surgery by looking at the temporal and nasal sclera for slightly whiter arcuate areas where recession or resection has been performed. For a medium angle of squint only the affected eye has surgery. For a larger angle, and for convergence excess, both eyes have surgery. Esotropias are usually slightly under-corrected and exotropia over-corrected, to avoid a later exotropia in both cases. Intermittent heterotropias have the deviation corrected exactly, to facilitate binocular control. A partially accommodative strabismus would normally have only the non-accommodative element surgically corrected, to facilitate binocular

Table 2.1 Orthoptic synonyms.

Appropriate term	Synonyms
Heterotropia	Strabismus, manifest deviation, decompensated deviation, squint
Heterophoria	Latent strabismus, latent deviation, latent squint
Esophoria	Latent convergence
Exophoria	Latent divergence
Convergence insufficiency	Convergence deficit, poor NPC
Convergence weakness	Near exotropia, convergence insufficiency
Convergence excess	Near esotropia, non-accommodative excess (a correct description where the AC/A ratio is low)
Divergence insufficiency	Divergence weakness, distance esotropia
Divergence excess	Distance exotropia
Microtropia	Monofixation syndrome, monofixational esophoria, retinal slip, fixation disparity, micro-strabismus, fusional disparity
Dissociated vertical deviation	DVD, dissociated vertical divergence, alternating hyperphoria, double hyperphoria, anaphoria, alternating sursumduction (in fact, this is one type of DVD; the other is alternating deorsumduction)
Paresis	Palsy, partial paralysis
Paralysis	Palsy, total paralysis
Relative vergences	Fusional reserves, prism vergences, fusion amplitudes, amplitudes
Decompensated heterophoria	Uncompensated heterophoria, heterophoria showing an associated phoria ('fixation disparity')

control. In paresis, surgery is usually delayed until several months have elapsed from the onset, so that any change in the direction of concomitance may occur. During this time treatment to avoid diplopia and contracture may be given. Surgery will have the aim of producing binocular vision ahead, and for downwards gaze, the areas of primary importance to the patient.

Where a substantial under-correction results, further surgery may be carried out on the opposite eye, or muscle, bearing in mind the 2-month period during which the deviation stabilizes.

Weakening of the action of an extra-ocular muscle is achieved by recession, tenotomy, myectomy or marginal myotomy. A recession detaches the muscle and re-inserts it further back (usually 5–9 mm) on the globe. A tenotomy sections a tendon, such as the superior oblique, or the lateral rectus in gross exotropia. In a myectomy the weakening is achieved by the removal of a section of the muscle. To weaken the effect of a muscle in its primary field of action (for the contralateral synergist of a paretic muscle, for example), a posterior fixation suture is used. This will not affect the balance of binocular control in other directions of gaze.

Strengthening of a muscle is achieved by resection, advancement, tucking or transplantation. A resection shortens a muscle, and re-attaches the shortened muscle to the original insertion. An advancement can be used to correct an excessive recession; tucking folds and thus shortens a muscle; and transplantation is used to bring strips of the superior and inferior rectus to the insertion of a paralysed lateral rectus.

2.3   The development of orthoptic techniques

Strabismus treatment is mentioned in the Ebers papyrus of c. 1600 BC, and in the writings of Hippocrates (450 BC).

Classical period AD 1500–1800

The use of face masks with perforations to encourage straightening of the eyes was advocated (Paré in 1530; Bartisch in 1583). The fact that squint is usually unilateral was noted by Buffon. The cover test was described (St. Ives in 1722). The precursor of the fusion training stereoscope was used by a general practitioner, Erasmus Darwin (1780), the grandfather of Charles Darwin.

The Victorian period

The first strabismus operation was devised, medial rectus myotomy (Dieffenbach in 1839). This resulted in consecutive exotropia in most cases, unless the myotomy was incomplete, or the muscle happened to re-attach more posteriorly. The horopter and its abnormal forms were described (Müller in 1840). Anomalous retinal correspondence (von Graefe in 1855) and its use of areas rather than points was discovered (Panum in 1859). The cover test was rediscovered, and accommodative strabismus explained as a failure of relative vergence control under the stress of excessive accommodative demand (Donders in 1864).

Exercises to improve relative vergences, together with stereoscope training and surgery were advocated in 1865 by Javal, who is sometimes called 'the father of orthoptics'. His 'bar reader' utilized physiological diplopia. Javal's work influenced the development of 'fusion tubes', used together with spectacles and surgery (Priestly-Smith in 1896). At the turn of the century Duane classified motor anomalies in terms of convergence and divergence excess, and insufficiency. Duane described the prism cover test and the retraction syndrome.

Twentieth century: to 1939

Sensory anomalies were graded as (i) simultaneous perception, (ii) fusion, (iii) stereopsis (Worth in 1903). This is a useful starting point, although it is possible to have stereopsis with a constant strabismus in anomalous correspondence. Remy introduced the diploscope, and prescribed exercises based on teaching the recognition of diplopia. The improvement of fusional amplitudes, by voluntary control exercises, was further developed (Cantonnet in 1920).

Outside France, exercises for squint were not thought worthwhile. However, the optometric London Refraction Hospital (now the Institute of Optometry) which opened in 1922 acquired orthoptic apparatus and gave exercises. An orthoptic clinic was organized there by Walter Green, the inventor of the synoptophore. This prompted Maddox (of rod, wing and double prism fame) to consider using non-medical assistance for orthoptic training. He trained his daughter Mary Maddox. She opened a private practice in London in 1928. Next year she was invited to open the first squint department in an ophthalmic hospital, the Royal Westminster. The British Orthoptic Society was formed in 1937 and a year later the American Orthoptic Council, thus creating the orthoptic profession, which is currently achieving graduate status in the UK.

Twentieth century: from 1939

The therapeutic difficulties arising from the late diagnosis of amblyopia was tackled by the use of pleoptic techniques (Bangerter, 1941; Cüppers, 1956). These techniques are still useful for neglected amblyopia. Anomalous correspondence was unveiled to its full extent in most squinters (Bagolini in 1958; Mallett in 1960). 'Monofixation syndrome' was described (Eustis and Parks in 1961) and re-defined more widely as microtropia (Lang in 1968). From 1962–1970 the work of Hubel and Wiesel has demonstrated the sensitive period in visual development.

The enthusiasm for orthoptic exercises declined from the 1960s with the realization that sensory and motor adaptations were too deeply ingrained in many squinters to be changed other than by surgery. However, American surgeons (e.g. Burian and von Noorden) have brought a degree of balance preferring conservative therapy: refractive correction, bifocals, negative additions and prisms, together with fusion exercises, for intermittent and accommodative strabismus, but amblyopia treatment followed by surgery for less plastic anomalies. Electro-physiological changes in amblyopia have been recorded (Arden, 1980). The need for early intervention in binocular anomalies is seen (Blakemore in 1974; Ikeda and Wright in 1975), and trials of early correction of refractive errors are in progress (Atkinson and Braddick in 1989).

Optometric contributions

The work of Cantonnet, in particular the use of 'mental effort' i.e. voluntary control of vergence, was applied with enthusiasm at the London Refraction

Hospital. Hospital staff produced textbooks on orthoptics (Giles in 1943; Gibson in 1945) and a history of orthoptics which included current clinical techniques (Revell, 1971). Other refraction hospitals were set up in Yorkshire and Scotland as the result of optometric enthusiasm. The Opticians Act 1958 stimulated the formation of the Orthoptic Association, currently the Orthoptic and Binocular Vision Association. The Act [section 25 (1)(d)] provides for rules to be made prohibiting or regulating the practice of orthoptics by ophthalmic and dispensing opticians, bodies corporate and their employees. Following submissions to the General Optical Council by the Faculty of Ophthalmologists, The British Optical Association and the Orthoptic Association, a decision was taken not to pass any rules. The Act also provides for the referral of patients suffering from an injury or disease of the eye to a registered medical practitioner for advice and treatment except in an emergency, or where the optician is providing treatment under section 25 (1)(d). Under the 1989 Act, this is section 31 (1)(d).

In general optometric practice, therapeutic advances have been made in:

1   The use of real space for orthoptic training (Lindsay in 1954).
2   Treating the confusion of vergence with version movements in squinters, and the use of physiological diplopia with small light sources and coloured filters (Calder Gillie in 1954).
3   The invention of the single mirror haploscope (Earnshaw in 1956) which gives an uninterrupted view of the patient's eyes and does not suffer from the small field of view, reduced illumination and proximal convergence of the synoptophore.
4   Techniques of physiological diplopia for home exercises using vertical line targets and wire reading (Earnshaw in 1960).
5   The development of a technique for monocular visual assessment under binocular viewing conditions (Humphriss in 1960).
6   Treating medium degrees of anomalous retinal correspondence by changing fixation to the deviated eye by fogging and prism correction of the deviation (Revell in 1969, based on the Walraven technique, see Kramer, 1949).
7   The use of transferred after-images to facilitate amblyopia treatment in teenagers (Caloroso in 1972).
8   The Bradford set of stereograms (Pickwell and Stockwell in 1970).
9   Contributions to the further development of physiological diplopia and other orthoptic techniques, and a textbook on Anomalies of Binocular Vision (Pickwell in 1984, 1989).
10 The recognition of fixation disparity as an indicator of stress on the vergence system (Mallett in 1964, 1966, 1974).
11 Methods of retinal correspondence measurement, and the treatment of amblyopia and nystagmus (Mallett in 1970, 1988).
12 The use of polarized vectograms and other orthoptic techniques by Vodnoy and other US practitioners (see Schor and Ciuffreda, 1983).

The current state of optometric practice includes diagnosis of anomalies of binocular vision, the treatment of the more amenable disorders, and the referral of most cases of strabismus, unless previously discharged for optometric care. A small number of practitioners and clinics take referred cases and acquire the expertise necessary for teaching and examining in this important subject. The prevalence of strabismus does not appear to have altered significantly over the years. This situation will only be improved by closer teamwork between the surveillance, diagnostic and management services provided by health visitors, general practitioners, optometrists, orthoptists and ophthalmologists.

CHAPTER 3
Ocular Deviations: Motor Anomalies

3.1   Introduction

Orthophoria is regarded as the normal binocular motor status. In sleep and general anaesthesia the eyes tend to diverge and elevate − this is also true of patients with non-restrictive esotropia. The average state of heterophoria in the general population, using a Maddox rod, is 1.4^{Δ} esophoria. Clinically compensated heterophoria may exceed the common range: 2^{Δ} exophoria to 4^{Δ} esophoria and up to 0.5^{Δ} of hyperphoria. Orthophoria does not describe the state of binocular vision in normal vision: it means parallel visual axes when the eyes are dissociated for clinical investigation. It is therefore rare.

Horizontal deviations are recorded as esophoria, esotropia, exophoria or exotropia. In writing to a general practitioner the convention was to use the terms latent or manifest, convergent or divergent squint. But GPs are quite able to look up the meaning of medical terms. It is best to restrict the use of 'convergence' and 'divergence' to vergence defects such as convergence insufficiency. The term 'strabismus' is the latin medical name for heterotropia and is currently used in writing; 'squint' is used in speech. Older orthoptists may refer to exophoria and esophoria as latent divergence and latent convergence respectively. Similarly the use of the biblical term 'palsy', though widespread, should ideally be replaced by the scientific terms 'paresis' for a partial paralysis, or 'paralysis' if complete.

There is a convention to record a vertical heterophoria as a right or left hyperphoria. When a hypotropia is intermittent or only becomes a hypotropia in some directions of gaze it is then appropriate to refer to a right or left intermittent hypotropia.

Ocular deviations may be concomitant (USA 'comitant') − equal in degree in all directions of gaze; or incomitant − varying in angle of deviation in different directions of gaze, clinically where the angle varies by more than 10^{Δ}. Incomitant deviations may be congenital, such as V and A patterns (or 'phenomena'), or acquired. Their origin may be neurological, for example nerve damage or neural hypoplasia, restrictive such as Duane's syndrome, or myogenic as in myasthenia gravis.

16

3.2   Aetiology of motor anomalies

Accommodative deviations are clearly responses of the optomotor reflex system — the child accommodates to overcome the blur produced by hypermetropia and becomes unable to maintain the demand for fusional divergence required to maintain normal binocular vision. This loss of control occurs when the child is tired or ill and is usually intermittent at first. Constant esotropia produces diplopia and confusion. The normal function of suppression, i.e. of physiological diplopia, is extended to remove the embarrassment caused by the deviated eye. Later, other adaptations, both sensory and motor, develop and tend to perpetuate the deviation. For example, hypertrophy of the medial rectus may occur. In addition, an abnormal motor correspondence develops to maintain a small, constant squint angle. So what was a fully accommodative squint becomes partially accommodative.

A *partially accommodative squint* may be partly due to refractive error and partly to muscle insertion anomalies.

A *non-accommodative squint* may be due to congenital muscle insertion anomalies. Delayed development of the lateral rectus muscles is another cause. This produces the rather uncommon 'cross-fixation' esotropia. The history is that 'both eyes used to turn in'. In fact there is a binocular zone centrally but the right eye fixates for left gaze. The left eye fixates for right gaze, (see Fig. 3.1). A similar effect is seen in a bilateral Duane's syndrome (type A or B). Depending on

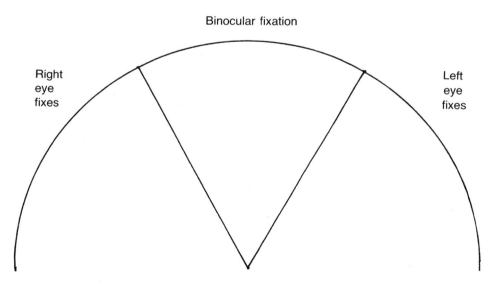

Fig. 3.1 The tripartite field of fixation in cross-fixation esotropia, and in bilateral Duane's syndrome (diagrammatic).

the speed of development of the lateral recti, especially towards the critical age of 6 months, when the cerebral cortex is taking over from sub-cortical reflex control, the patient may have esophoria, intermittent esotropia, unilateral esotropia or alternating esotropia.

A momentary esotropia or exotropia may be seen in babies in the first 6 months of life but this should not become frequent or persistent. A diary should be kept by the parents and the occurrence of heterotropia should decline from 3 months, when the vergence system starts to operate and stereopsis develops.

Intermittent exotropias have recently been reported in 50% of babies up to 6 months old. After this age such a finding is abnormal. *Exodeviations* found in adult life develop as exophoria in the first year of life, gradually become intermittent exotropia and in 50% of cases constant exotropia. The aetiology of exodeviations may be a combination of anatomic and neural factors. Abnormal muscle insertions, orbital shape or check ligaments may be present. Abnormal optomotor control may be due to a deficit in convergence innervation or a faulty interaction between convergence and divergence control.

Vertical deviations have been classified by Bielschowsky (1938) as:

1 concomitant;
2 paretic;
3 due to unilateral inferior oblique overaction (elevation in adduction − the commonest incomitancy), (see 8.3);
4 dissociated vertical divergence: alternating sursumduction if either eye moves upward when covered, deorsumduction if either eye moves downward;
5 vertical deviations combined with other deviations.

Classification aids understanding and management of these deviations. However, most medical conditions show a continuum or spectrum of anomalies ranging from the slight to the severe. So there are many intermediate and overlapping conditions. Heterophoria may become decompensated and as control worsens the condition may be described as an intermittent strabismus. There is a type of squint which occurs on alternate days (cyclic esotropia) which may gradually become a constant esotropia. Another progression might involve a compensated heterophoria which becomes decompensated in the direction of action of one extra-ocular muscle, next a paretic squint, complete paralysis and finally a restrictive squint with fibrosis of the involved muscle. Finally there is the group of intermediate deviations known as microtropia.

Microtropia (synonyms: monofixation syndrome, monofixational heterophoria) is a stable form of deviation which is intermediate between heterophoria and heterotropia, (see 7.13). Microtropia includes a range of micro-deviations with varying motor and sensory adaptations. Microtropia is defined differently by different authors. Von Noorden's classic discussion of microtropia (1985) should be read, together with recent papers by Eustis and Parks (1989) and Jampolsky (1989).

3.3 Eye movement systems

There are five systems of eye movement:

1 Fixation system: the patient is asked to look at a target, or reflexly does so.
2 (Slow) pursuit system: as in the motility test and the slow phase of optokinetic nystagmus. Velocity is 30°/second.
3 Saccadic system: the patient is asked to look from one target laterally or vertically to another. It also mediates the fast phase of optokinetic nystagmus and the fast phase of vestibular nystagmus. The saccadic system is typically used in reading lines of print. The velocity is 700°/second. There are also micro-saccades which maintain fixation.
4 Vergence system: as in convergence, divergence, vertical vergence (5^Δ vertical fusional amplitude) and cyclovergence (5^Δ cyclofusional reserves). The velocity is 20°/second.
5 Non-optic reflex eye movements: initiated by the vestibular reflex and tonic neck reflex. Also Bell's phenomenon, which causes the eyes to deviate up and out upon forced lid opening while the patient attempts to keep his eyes closed. The velocity is 300°/second. Proprioceptive feedback is also derived from the extra-ocular muscles and used to maintain eye position (Hansen, 1988).

3.4 Vergence system anomalies

Heterophorias and heterotropias, which are here collectively called deviations are defects of the vergence system of eye movement. They may be precipitated by local factors within the orbit or by refractive errors. Pareses are defects of individual muscle motor function and may be caused by lesions of the medial longitudinal fasciculus, the cerebral nerve nuclei, the nerves or of the muscles (see Table 3.1). Other anomalies of eye movement such as nystagmus may also occur either separately or associated with deviations and pareses, as in internuclear ophthalmoplegia, (see 9.1).

3.5 Fixation disparity and prism adaptation

Fixation disparity can be regarded as: (i) a trigger to fusional vergence and (ii) a symptom of stress on the vergence eye movement system (Mallett, 1964). The limit of the binocular response to fixation disparity is a combination of the amplitude of Panum's area (which itself varies with target size, illumination and

Table 3.1 Summary of neurological eye movement disorders.

Defect	Lesion	Mechanism
1. Loss of movement in field of action of affected muscle	Damage to nucleus or nerve III IV or VI	Vergence, pursuit fixation, saccadic
2(a). Loss of voluntary eye movement in affected direction: 'gaze paresis'	Frontal: area 8 lesion	Saccadic
2(b). Oculogyric crisis. Erratic and involuntary saccadic eye movements	Occipital and descending pathways, e.g. measles encephalitis	Fixation reflex
3. Internuclear ophthalmoplegia: gaze paresis to affected side, nystagmus to opposite side	Medial longitudinal fasciculus: e.g. lesion adjacent to VI and VIII nuclei and paramedian pontine reticular formation	Saccadic, pursuit
4. Loss of reflex and voluntary movements to one side	Pontine gaze centre	Saccadic, pursuit, vestibular
5. Overshoot in motility test (dysmetria). Ocular flutter: short bursts of horizontal saccades	Cerebellum, e.g. brain damage at birth. Senile changes	Saccadic, pursuit Saccadic
6. Loss of saccades which are replaced by slow eye movements	Progressive supranuclear degeneration, Huntington's chorea	Saccadic
7. Jerky motility: saccades superimposed upon pursuit movement: 'cogwheeling'	Interruption of pathways between the occipital lobes and the pontine gaze centre	Saccadic

These anomalies are discussed in Chapter 9.

speed of binocular vergence movements), along with the amount of suppression and the state of retinal correspondence. A full discussion can be found in *'Vergence Eye Movements'* (Schor and Ciuffreda, 1983). The amount of prism required to align the nonius marks on a Mallett fixation disparity test is called the 'associated phoria', because it is measured while the eyes are still associated, i.e. not dissociated (see 6.7).

There is a close relationship between esophoria and an indication of decompensated esophoria on a fixation disparity test ('eso-slip'). Exo-slip does not always accompany exophoria and eso-slip may even appear, showing over-compensation. Neither does the presence of fixation disparity always warrant the treatment of the associated phoria, unless symptoms are also present. However, in children the absence of symptoms may be due to suppression, in which case treatment may be desirable. If treatment is not given the suppression may deepen into amblyopia. Alternatively, the decompensation may become worse, and symptoms of discomfort, or diplopia may follow. At the least the child should be monitored every few months. It has been suggested that even in non-symptomatic adults, job performance may be enhanced by correcting heterophoria which appears decompensated on a fixation disparity test (Mallett, 1974).

The normal state of heterophoria in the general population is $1.4^\triangle$ esophoria (von Noorden, 1985). In optometric patients the average heterophoria appears to be $1^\triangle$ exophoria in the author's experience. Taking this as normal there seems to be what might be called an 'orthophorization' process, analogous to emmetro-pization. However, some individuals with phorias return to the initial phoria despite the interposition of sizeable amounts of 'correcting' prism. In these cases the benefit of prescribing prism may be based on the effect on symptoms, or on prism adaptation methods.

The amount of heterophoria can vary during and following the wearing of prisms. It has been shown that an initial *associated phoria* of, say, $6^\triangle$ produced by placing a prism in front of an orthophoric patient halves in 3.5 minutes: *prism adaptation* (North and Henson, 1981; North *et al.*, 1990). The associated phoria is the amount of prism required to align the monocular polarized bars on a Mallett fixation disparity test.

In European optometric practice it has become conventional to refer to the associated phoria as 'the fixation disparity'. This is because the associated phoria is measured on a fixation disparity unit. In this text the correct term 'associated phoria' will be used for accuracy.

With the American Sheedy Disparometer it is possible to adjust physically the monocular bars to remove an apparent misalignment; this measures the actual fixation disparity. However this does not correlate as well for symptom relief as the associated phoria. A further assessment of binocular motor control can be made by plotting fixation disparity curves by using a Sheedy Disparometer, or by modifying a Mallett unit physically to move the nonius bars to produce an apparent alignment to the patient. The Zeiss Polartest also utilizes fixation disparity for prescribing prisms, or modifying the refractive correction.

Absence of prism adaptation is an indicator for prescribing prism: the associated phoria disappears even after 3.5 minutes of wearing a trial prism. This is useful for exophoria where the initial 'fixation disparity' i.e. associated phoria (or lack of it) is not always reliable as an indicator of clinical need for phoria management. There the initial associated phoria should be taken with an arbitrary amount of correcting prism, say 1^Δ initially, and the fixation disparity test used to re-measure the associated phoria at 3.5 minutes. If the associated phoria has not returned to the initial reading pre-prism the indication is that, if symptoms are present, the patient is unable to prism adapt and requires either prism or exercises or refractive control of the deviation, or a combination of these. Fresnel lenses may be used for a trial of prisms, but they are not cheap and it is usually better to get the prism right the first time.

Because a symptom-free patient can easily adapt to various amounts of prism this does not mean that prisms have no therapeutic effect in symptomatic heterophoria. But it is possible to prescribe the correcting prism for both distance and near even though the decompensation occurs at only one working distance. The patient needs the prism for one working distance, and adapts to it for the other.

Thus prism controlled bifocals or bi-prism lenses which in the past may have been considered essential will not be required in many instances. In fact it can be quite disturbing to go from one area of a lens without prism to another with prism − even if clinically indicated. The intriguing idea of prescribing a variable prism is not practicable as a prism which steadily increases in power across its surface is normally described as a negative cylinder! (Fig. 3.2). For some cases of paresis, however, serial strips of Fresnel prisms of increasing power have been used.

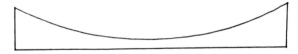

Fig. 3.2 A variable power prism (a cylinder).

A new protocol, which is still being developed, for prescribing prisms using 'prism adaptation' is as follows:

1 Measure phoria at 6 m, by Maddox rod or prism cover test.
2 Measure associated phoria, by Mallett fixation disparity test (the amount of prism to align the nonius marks).
3 Put this prism up in front of one eye.
4 Wait 3 minutes. Re-measure associated phoria.
5 If the second measurement of the associated phoria is now zero, prescribe prism equal to the original associated phoria, split equally between each eye. The patient has 'soaked up' the prism and needs it to avoid decompensation.
6 If the second measurement of the associated phoria is greater than zero, fixation disparity is still present but the patient does not soak up the prism and can cope without it under the test conditions at the time.

7 If (6) applies, but the patient has symptoms, perhaps when tired or at work, remove the prism (3 above). Put up $2^\triangle$ adverse prism (e.g. base-in for esophoria). Wait 3 minutes. Measure the associated phoria again. If the associated phoria at this point is greater than zero, the patient cannot cope with the adverse prism. The symptoms are probably due to decompensation. Prescribe half the first measurement (at 2 above) of the associated phoria. Review in 1 month.

8 Alternatives to prescribing prisms should be considered. These include changes in the patient's general and working conditions, orthoptic exercises, and modifying the refractive correction, (see Chapter 6).

CHAPTER 4
Ocular Adaptations: Sensory Anomalies

4.1 Introduction

When the object of binocular fixation is imaged on the fovea of one eye and an area of peripheral retina of the other eye, that is on disparate retinal areas, the object is projected and seen in two different directions. This is called *diplopia*. The patient may describe what he sees as double vision. The simultaneous arrival in the visual cortex of different images from each fovea is called *confusion*. If the object is a single, small, bright, test light the observer is more likely to report double vision. Where the object of regard is the normal complex scene of a familiar room or view, the observer is more likely to report confusion: 'everything goes into one'. Conversely, a report of double vision may indicate merely an out of focus ghost image around the object of regard, and not a binocular anomaly at all.

The first sensory response to a loss of binocular motor or sensory co-ordination will be a reduction in stereoscopic acuity. Stereopsis has been described as the thermometer of binocular vision. Reduced stereopsis usually indicates abnormal suppression. Exceptionally, reduced stereopsis may apparently exist without other binocular or monocular anomalies. Clinically, an early indicator of an intermittent squint may be seen in failure to pass the Lang stereopsis test. This test can be used on children as young as 8 months old with a high degree of success. On older children an abnormal finding on a fixation disparity test, such as displacement or suppression of a nonius bar, is an indication of a binocular vision problem. As the original intermittent deviation becomes a constant squint, so the associated suppression changes from a facultative to an obligatory state and then proceeds to the monocular anomaly of amblyopia. It is important to record the suppression test used and to use more than one test (see 4.4).

Together with the appearance of suppression the retinal correspondence is suspended. Small errors in conjugate eye movement control can occur without spoiling binocularity due to the flexibility inherent in Panum's fusional areas. This allows misalignment of peripheral (15°) retinal areas by 60″ between the two eyes without confusion or diplopia, and 15″ centrally (see von Noorden, 1985). In the case of strabismus, Panum's fusional areas enlarge peripherally and thus allow a degree of binocular perception. The retinal correspondence is however abnormal. Anomalous retinal correspondence ('ARC') spreads fovealward and is probably a function of the cortical association areas; Brodmann's area 19. Eventually only two areas each subtending 1 or 2 degrees (at the fixation spot and at the fovea of the deviated eye) may remain as suppression areas, being unable to correspond abnormally with the fixating eye.

Despite being a binocular anomaly, ARC may revert to normal retinal correspondence ('NRC') if fixation is switched to the usually deviated eye. This suggests a link between motor and sensory adaptations. Following the development of suppression, or ARC, are the monocular adaptations of amblyopia and eccentric fixation. Of course, the deviated eye can hardly be said to fixate (under binocular conditions) either centrally or eccentrically, since this function defaults to the fixing eye except on extreme lateral eye movement to the side of the deviated eye, in its monocular field. Nevertheless, on covering the fixing eye, the fixation characteristics of the deviated eye can be checked.

The classical 'grades of binocular vision' formulated by Worth were: (i) simultaneous perception; (ii) fusion; (iii) stereopsis. A more helpful classification is to note the extent of diplopia, suppression and anomalous retinal correspondence. The majority of squints show ARC with small suppression areas at the fovea and the point receiving the fixation image in the deviated eye.

4.2   Stereopsis

Stereopsis is a sensitive test of binocularity. Three dimensional tests are difficult to use; for example the Frisby stereotest (Fig. 4.1) will produce monocular clues to depth perception if it, or the patient's head, is moved or if a shadow moves across the test plate. Two dimensional stereotests are designed to present different images to each eye. The TNO stereotest (Fig. 4.2) uses red and green glasses and random dot anaglyph stereopairs varying from 2000″ to 15″. The absence of tests between 2000″ and 480″ can be compensated partly by varying the test distance. By holding the TNO test book at twice the normal test distance the stereo-disparities are halved so that the 2000″ test becomes 1000″. The cross polarized Randot (Fig. 4.3) is an update of the Wirt Fly Test (Fig. 4.4) but, unlike the TNO, the Randot test is a combination of random dot and monocularly visible targets. A normal result of 20″ is roughly equivalent to the difficulty of seeing 60″ on the TNO test.

Both TNO and Randot tests require the patient to wear glasses. However the random dot Lang test provides different images to each eye without glasses and has no monocular clues. It can therefore be used with children as young as 6 months old when convergence and fixation on to each of the three targets in turn will be seen in a high proportion of normal babies. At 9 months most babies will attempt to grasp the test objects. Despite the test stereo-disparities

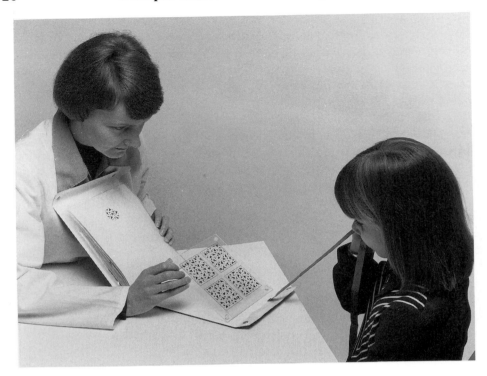

Fig. 4.1 The Frisby stereotest.

ranging only between 1200″ and 550″ — quite gross — such responses probably rule out the presence of significant amblyopia, anisometropia in excess of two dioptres, suppression, squint, a central scotoma as in Stargardt's disease and major deficits of accommodation and convergence (Lang, 1988). In particular the conditions creating an intermittent squint are likely to cause failure on this test, *even while the eyes are not deviated.* The Lang test is in effect a test of visual acuity and ametropia. Thus a dubious result with the Lang test requires repetition of the test at the next visit and adequate investigation to explain the cause of the poor response. Failure to carry out a cycloplegic refraction coupled with a negative Lang test would not be acceptable because any finding of reduced visual function requires further action. In deviations which vary with fixation distance (e.g. divergence excess) it is possible to have stereopsis for near, but not for distance fixation. Distance stereopsis requires a projected stereotest. However, a distance fixation disparity test will often show the suppression associated with a reduction in stereopsis.

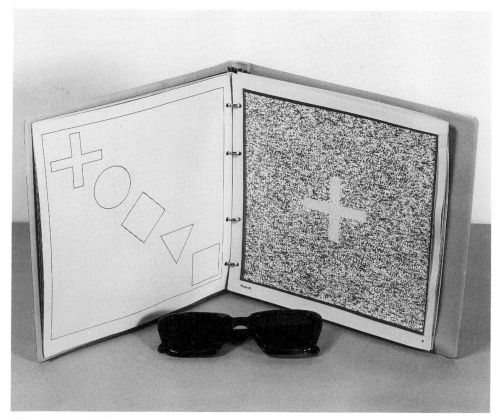

Fig. 4.2 The TNO stereotest.

4.3   Diplopia

The classification of binocular diplopia is as follows:

1   Physiological diplopia: normally the patient is unaware of this. Occasionally, having discovered it, a child may find it difficult to ignore and may present with physiological diplopia as a symptom.
2   Pathological diplopia with NRC, (non-paretic), e.g. secondary squint following a traumatic cataract in children of 8 years or older.
3   Pathological diplopia with NRC and paresis, e.g. due to an intra-cranial space occupying lesion.
4   Pathological diplopia with unharmonious ARC
    (i) 'paradoxical': the pre-operative ARC continues unchanged post-operatively, instead of adjusting to the post-operative squint angle

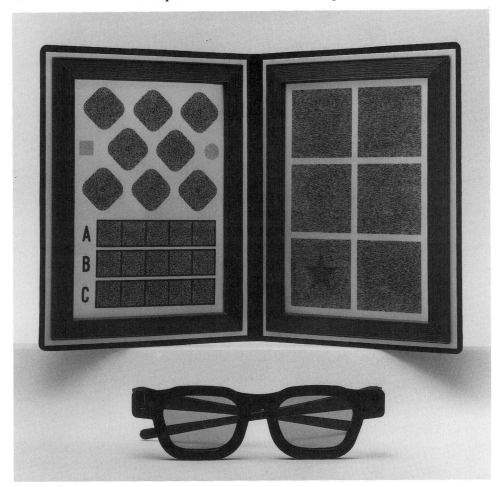

Fig. 4.3 The Randot stereotest.

(ii)   binocular triplopia (= 'monocular diplopia'): pre-operative ARC per-
         sists post-operatively, and the innate NRC re-appears post-operatively.
         This is rare, but can be induced experimentally or for ARC treatment.

If diplopia is of paretic origin, the patient generally will attempt to remove
diplopia by moving his head in the direction of the affected muscle. Older
patients may need to be taught this, once treatment of the underlying cause has
been started. In incomitant squint, diplopia will be intermittent at first when
the child is tired. There may be a history of unilateral eye closure or covering
and falling or clumsiness.
     It is helpful, in cases of diplopia, to plot the zone over which double vision is

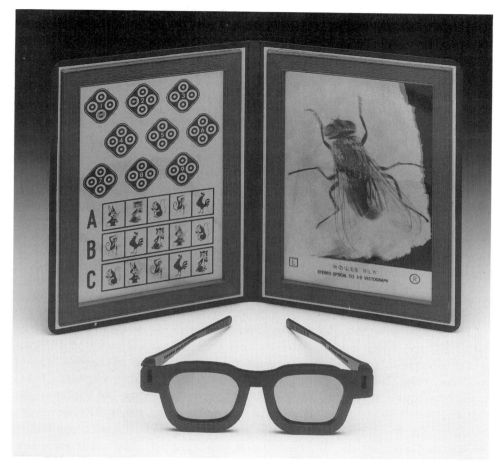

Fig. 4.4 The Wirt stereotest.

seen; the diplopia field. The amount of vertical and horizontal prism required to eliminate diplopia in each of the nine cardinal directions of gaze should also be recorded, in the form of a 'diplopia matrix' (see 5.11). The patient should be reviewed from time to time to note changes in the diplopia fields and the diplopia matrix.

The *management* of diplopia is generally that of the underlying motor and sensory anomalies present. In intractable diplopia, some patients are able to ignore one image. In other cases, this is only possible if one image is degraded by hypnotic suggestion, by partial occlusion (e.g. Fablon, Contact, Blenderm semi-occluding membranes), or by a grossly defocussed contact lens. Rarely, cases of diplopia-phobia occur. These may require complete occlusion of the binocular visual field of one eye. This can be achieved by wearing a scleral contact lens which is totally occluding except for a temporal zone to allow vision in the monocular (temporal) field of vision, for safety reasons.

Some patients prefer to retain diplopia if low grade depth perception is still possible, e.g. for pouring liquids. In these cases one image should be degraded optically, to avoid the confusing effect of two clear images. Diplopia and a degree of depth perception are not totally incompatible. This state occurs physiologically both in front and behind the normal horopter. For the management of diplopia in unharmonious ARC see 4.7.

The causes of monocular diplopia (in order of frequency) are as follows:

1   Lenticular abnormalities e.g. cataract.
2   Uncorrected or wrongly corrected astigmatism.
3   Corneal abnormalities e.g. keratoconus.
4   Retinal abnormalities e.g. macular oedema.
5   Visual cortex abnormalities: central diplopia as in certain occipital cortex lesions, and also in hysterical conversion, (patient may be having treatment for anxiety and depression).
6   Post-operative 'monocular diplopia' (see above).

Post-operative monocular diplopia, due to the presence post-operatively of both NRC and ARC, is more correctly described as *binocular triplopia*. If, post-operatively, there is a small residual esotropia, the fixing eye will see the fixation point correctly, and the deviating eye may see two more images, one using NRC at the new squint angle and one using ARC derived from the old squint angle. Usually, both NRC and the old ARC are suppressed and a new ARC develops, providing the deviation remains stable and the operation is carried out before the age of 8 years or so. A recurrence of this condition may occur for a few hours or days under exceptional circumstances. In one case, it was associated with the death of the mother of a 10-year-old girl. ARC can be regarded as a correspondence between the fixating fovea and the fixation point in the deviated eye. Thus post-operatively in the typical esotropia where the angle is reduced but not completely eliminated (to avoid consecutive exotropia), the ARC slides across from the old to the new fixation point, closer to the deviated fovea. This type of adjustment is confirmed by findings that on a synoptophore some ARC patients can maintain gross fusion while the tubes are moved, although their eyes do not move (von Noorden, 1985). A fluid form of ARC is also thought to be present in some paretic squints.

The onset of diplopia, together with its duration, frequency and direction — oblique, vertical or horizontal — should be noted. Is there is an A or a V pattern? Where intermittent diplopia is reported, but not found on examination, see Table 4.1.

Table 4.1 Double vision check list (for use by patients with occasional diplopia).

1. Does the double vision go when you cover:
   (i) the right eye?
   (ii) the left eye?

2. In which 'Union Jack' direction of gaze is the double vision the greatest, excluding the vertical direction?

3. Which eye do you have to cover to remove the furthest image horizontally or vertically?

4.4   Suppression

Once an eye has deviated in a child young enough to suppress readily, a difficult process after 8 years old, then the fixation image falling on the deviated retina will be suppressed, unless falling on the blind spot. A second suppression area will develop at the deviated fovea. (Where the fixation image falls on the blind spot, the squint has been termed 'the blind spot syndrome'. This is now felt to be a chance occurrence. The terminology should no longer be used.)

In infantile esotropia with cross fixation, suppression will transfer from one eye to the other, according to which eye is being used to fixate. Similarly, in adults with decompensated divergence excess, the suppression will alternate, depending upon whether the right or left field of vision is being used. Here the

Table 4.2 Tests for suppression.

Test or Instrument	Features
Lang stereotest	Random dot, no analysing glasses
TNO stereotest	Random dot, needs analysing glasses
Randot stereotest	Random dot, some monocular clues, needs polarized analysing glasses
Titmus stereotest	Monocular clues, needs polarized analysing glasses
Frisby stereotest	True stereopsis, no analysing glasses, but prone to give monocular clues due to parallax
Mallett fixation disparity test	Polarized nonius marks can produce suppression due to retinal rivalry, stereotest may require prism to aid fusion, suppression test useful but should be confirmed by using a separate stereotest
Holmes stereoscope with Bradford stereograms	Gross test, useful for children over 4 years

Table 4.2 Cont.

Test or Instrument	Features
Worth Four Dot test	This test consists of distance and near units with two white, one red and one green aperture, viewed with analysing red and green glasses or goggles. It is popular in orthoptic departments but is relatively crude and may produce false positive and negative results. For example, a suppression area may fall within the centre of the test, and miss all the apertures. The test produces retinal rivalry, which may cause false positive results
Synoptophore and similar haploscope instruments	The most crude form of suppression test is to use the lion and the cage slides for each eye. This is the most extreme form of retinal rivalry stimulation, and resulted in the historic assumption that most squinters had suppression alone rather than anomalous retinal correspondence with small suppression zones in the central retinal area (see 4.6). Less crude slides may be used, but the instrument suffers from proximal convergence, low illumination levels, and a grossly restricted field of view. The semi-silvered mirror option on the Stanworth synoptiscope removes most of these objections for suppression testing
Bagolini striated lens	See text
Bagolini red filter bar	Diplopia marks the end point
Four prism dioptre test	See text
Vertical prism test (to produce diplopia)	
Bar reading	
Convergence	If the line target moves to one side at the break point
Subjective cover test	Absence of diplopia in heterotropia when the cover is removed suggests suppression
Binocular visual acuity	May be less than monocular acuity in the presence of suppression
Contrast sensitivity	Shows a monocular reduction

whole of each retina is suppressed alternately (Cooper and Record, 1986). Complete suppression is also referred to (somewhat negatively) as 'lack of retinal correspondence'. Patients with large angle exotropias may acquire a habit of alternately suppressing each eye so that a kind of panoramic vision is attained rather like that in animals with wide eye separation (see Fig. 4.5).

The usual progression of suppression is for the two original suppression areas (at the fovea and the fixation point of the deviated eye) to join, covering

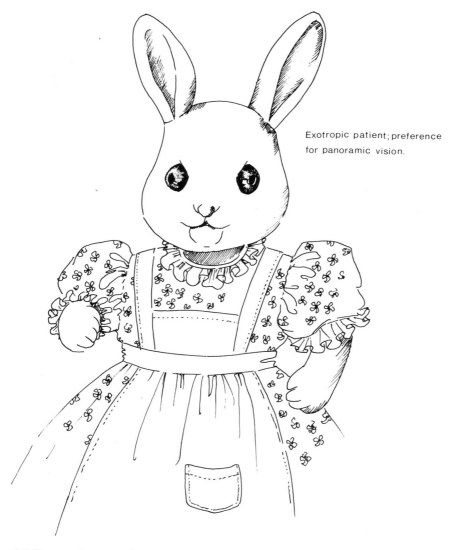

Exotropic patient; preference for panoramic vision.

Fig. 4.5 Panoramic exotropia.

perhaps an area of 30°. This is certainly the case in deep suppression. Suppression appears to be initiated cortically but possibly also has a retinal component. Suppression is not a process which involves the faculty of perception. However, many patients with long-standing diplopia can learn to *ignore* the fainter image successfully; a perceptual process.

4.5   Assessing suppression in squint

In heterotropia it is convenient to test for suppression using a grade two Bagolini lens and a neutral density filter bar. A Bagolini lens can be approximated by smearing a low power trial lens to produce a cylindrical streak from a small light source − ideally at 3 m and also at 33 cm. If a 6 m test distance is used it may be necessary to reduce slightly the level of room illumination, or to use a grade four Bagolini lens. The depth of suppression is measured by sliding a neutral density filter bar, graduated in log units, in increasing depth of absorption in front of the non-suppressing eye until a streak is seen by the other eye with a Bagolini lens in front of it. Alternatively, the patient may report diplopia when the suppression ceases. A suppression area at the fixation point of the deviated eye is indicated by a central gap in the Bagolini streak. In this case it is reasonable to suppose that there will also be a similar small suppression area at the fovea of the deviated eye. Even in the absence of a gap, any indication that one Bagolini streak is fainter than the other is an indication of suppression. The traditional test for suppression is the Worth Four Dot test. This may miss a small central suppression area or be entirely within a larger one, and therefore should not be used by the inexperienced.

4.6   Assessing suppression in heterophoria

In heterophoria suppression may be assessed by the loss of stereo-acuity. The TNO test is probably the most sensitive stereotest. Where the phoria decompensates intermittently, no stereo loss may be shown in an adult. Here it may be necessary to infer the change in visual function from symptoms and motor findings such as a high phoria. Inability to peg washing on a line using binocular vision is a symptom of reduced stereopsis, though also of incomitancy (A or V pattern for example).

Fixation disparity tests are frequently used in optometric practice to assess binocular function. For distance vision, reduction in intensity or disappearance of a monocular polarized marker indicates suppression. However, fixation disparity tests involve some retinal rivalry in that similar objects are not imaged on corresponding retinal areas, and supplementary tests such as acuity and stereopsis should be assessed before prescribing any treatment. For near vision the Mallett fixation disparity test includes a specific test for suppression and stereopsis. Prisms base-in may be needed to allow fusion on this stereopsis test. Consider lighting and working distance of both the test unit and of the patient in his own environment.

The *management* of suppression is described in 6.10 and 6.11.

4.7   Anomalous retinal correspondence

Anomalous retinal correspondence (ARC) is defined as a binocular condition in which the fovea of the fixing eye has a common visual direction (i.e. projection) with a non-foveal area of the deviating eye.

Development of ARC

ARC is believed to arise by the operation of the normal mechanism which suppresses physiological diplopia extending an area of suppression across the deviated retina until the image of the fixation object is located. At this point harmonious ARC operates. The original normal retinal correspondence (NRC) is simultaneously suppressed. If correspondence between the fixing fovea and any point between the deviated fovea and fixation point occurred, it would be unharmonious and accompanied by diplopia – a condition only found shortly after surgery, or briefly following a significant change in refractive or prismatic correction. The excellent review of ARC by Jennings (1985) should be read.

Conditions for development of ARC

1   Squint before 4 years old, especially before 30 months.
2   Delay in treatment.
3   Small constant squint angle.
4   Esotropia > exotropia.
5   Unilateral > alternating squint.

Thus early surgery with the usual intended under-correction is likely to provide the conditions for ARC to develop. The original NRC is suspended, although under experimental conditions its presence can be detected. There is a risk in fully accommodative squint, if the full cycloplegic refraction is not given. The previously large variable squint angle, altering with accommodative demand, may now become a small constant angle squint. The conditions are now ideal for ARC to develop, where before the variability of the squint angle ensured that suppression was the only adaptation possible. So what was a treatable deviation develops a deep ARC and becomes virtually untreatable. An under-correction of hypermetropia in strabismus may be accepted, provided it results in normal binocular fusion.

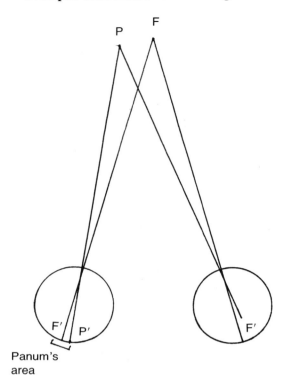

Fig. 4.6 Panum's fusional area. F, the fixation point; F', the fovea of each eye; P, a point adjacent to the fixation point; P', the retinal image of P. Objects imaged within the Panum's fusional area of one eye may be fused with the corresponding retinal element of the other eye. (Not to scale.)

ARC develops due to the enlargement of Panum's fusional areas (see Fig. 4.6). These normally range from 6″ to 10″ horizontally by two-thirds that dimension vertically in the foveal area, to 35″ to 45″ at 13° from the fovea. There is also some increase in size if the disparate images move apart more slowly across each retina as bifoveal function is lost. In strabismus these areas become much larger and have been called pseudo-Panum's areas. They are also larger peripherally and allow peripheral binocular perception in an early onset squint. This peripheral ARC is thought to spread fovealwards, replacing the initial large suppression area. Anomalous correspondence also explains the phenomenon of the deviated eye 'running before the prism' or increasing the squint angle when a correcting prism is applied (base-out for esotropia) except of course in patients shortly after squint onset, when prisms may produce bifoveal stimulation. However, peripheral fusion may also occur in patients with suppressed NRC.

In order for ARC (a sensory adaptation) to occur, there must develop an abnormal 'motor correspondence' (see 3.2). This must maintain the squint at a constant angle while the eyes make version, vergence and a combination of both these eye movements. Once established, abnormal motor correspondence like ARC tends to perpetuate the squint even if any refractive cause, such as hypermetropia, is corrected.

In an acute paresis it is the normal motor and sensory correspondence which produce disorientation and false projection even to the point of apparent movement of objects (try this by going cross-eyed) and diplopia. In microtropia, deeply ingrained anomalous correspondence and gross stereopsis are found (see 7.13).

Depending upon the degree of interference with binocular visual input, various tests for ARC may either detect or fail to detect ARC in a given patient. Bagolini striated lenses interfere least with binocular fusion, followed by the synoptophore and then after-image investigation (Fig. 4.7, and see Rutstein *et al.*, 1989).

The depth of adaptation (the measure of permanence) of ARC may be measured with a *neutral density filter bar*. A Bagolini striated lens is placed (so that the streak is seen at 90° to the direction of the deviation — vertically for a horizontal squint) before the deviated eye, together with the lightest step of the

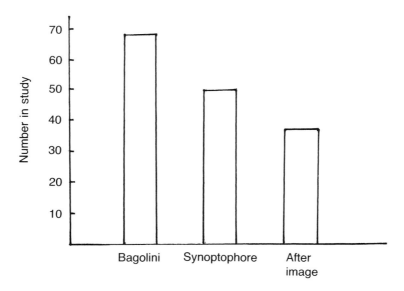

Fig. 4.7 The detection of ARC with tests of decreasing sensitivity. (After Rutstein, Daum and Eskridge, 'Clinical Characteristics of Anomalous Correspondence', *Optometry and Vision Science*, **66** 7 (July 1989).)

neutral density filter bar. The patient fixates a spot light at 3 or 6 m. The filter is increased until the streak seen by the deviated eye disappears. For an alternating strabismus, Bagolini lenses are placed in front of each eye, with axes at 45° and 135° respectively.

The neutral density bar result gives the depth of ARC in log units. These neutral density units ('ND') equal the reciprocal of log transmission of the filter. This gives an indication of prognosis. Under 0.6 ND log units some response to a major change in refractive correction, bifocals, prisms or exercises to establish fusional movement may be expected. Between 0.6 and 1.0 ND log units, response would only be to very determined anti-ARC treatment on a synopto-phore. Over 1.0 ND log units the ARC is probably best left alone or indeed encouraged both as a second best substitute for normal binocular vision and so that glasses may be removed later. Here the small angle squint is maintained even without refractive correction, by the deep ARC, thus avoiding diplopia.

Alternatively, the depth of ARC may be measured (at 40 cm) with the modified *Mallett Near Vision Fixation Disparity Unit*, which gives similar results to a Bagolini lens. A neutral density filter bar may be used to measure the point at which suppression of the nonius bar occurs. This gives the depth of ARC. The distance Mallett Fixation Disparity Test may also be used to assess ARC, but at a fixation distance of 150 cm. ARC can be measured with a synoptophore or by using monocular foveal after-images, but these methods will not detect the less deeply ingrained stages of ARC.

Subjective and objective angles of squint in ARC

The 'subjective angle' is the angular separation in subjective space between the fixing fovea and the fixation point in the deviated eye, especially when measured by the patient moving the tubes of a synoptophore (Fig. 4.8) to 'align' the two images. The 'objective angle' is the angle between the two foveas, especially when measured by the practitioner on a synoptophore by alternately occluding the image going to each eye and adjusting the angles of the tubes until no eye movement is seen. The 'angle of the anomaly' is the difference between the subjective and objective angles. If the angle of the anomaly differs from the squint angle measured by the prism cover test, it must be an artefact of synoptophore testing unless the patient also complains of diplopia in real space conditions, in which case a true unharmonious ARC may be present. Such artefacts are produced where there is a large central suppression area, or due to proximal convergence.

Management of ARC

ARC occurs mainly in partially accommodative strabismus, and its management is described in section 7.4. Other techniques available include:

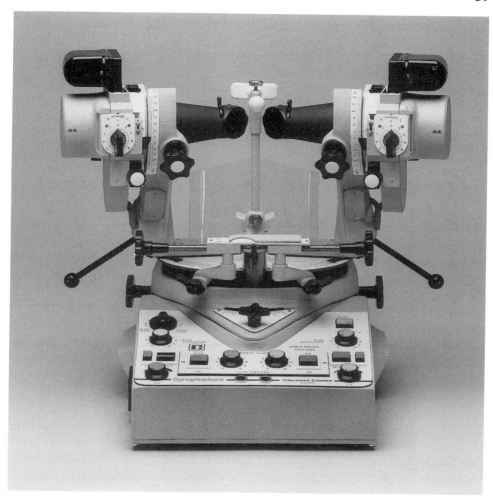

Fig. 4.8 The synoptophore. (Clement Clarke International: Model 2001).

1 *Physiological diplopia*, using the same technique as for treatment of suppression described in 6.10.

2 *Prisms* may be prescribed, 6^Δ base-up for one eye, and 6^Δ base-down for the other eye, and with the base directions reversed on alternate days; or with an adverse prism, say 15^Δ Fresnel prism base-in for esotropia (Mallett, 1979). These prisms produce suppression, which is one step closer to normal binocular vision, and thus easier to treat than ARC. The patient is being taken back along the path of abnormal adaptations which he has made: normal binocular single vision, diplopia, suppression and ARC. This technique also has the effect of improving cosmetic appearance as the eyes appear to be further apart.

3   A *synoptophore* may be used with the tubes set at the objective squint angle and simultaneous vision slides flashed alternately at 4 Hz before each eye for 20–40 minutes once or twice a week. The detail should be large enough for the amblyopic eye to see clearly.

Macular massage stimulates NRC by setting the tubes at the objective angle and moving the tube in front of the deviated eye laterally across the foveal region to stimulate the normal use of the fovea. ARC develops from the periphery. The foveal region adapts last or merely suppresses.

The *Stanworth synoptiscope* has semi-silvered mirrors and allows the patient to fixate a distant spotlight while the two tubes (set at the objective angle) are moved together laterally, to stimulate corresponding retinal areas: *kinetic stimulation*. It may also be used for other free space anti-ARC exercises (Mallett, 1970).

4   A *single mirror haploscope* (see 6.12) may be used in a similar manner to a synoptophore.

Often the effect of treatment may be to reduce the ARC depth, while relative vergences (fusional amplitudes) are improved. The ARC may not totally disappear, but continues to prevent the appearance of diplopia.

The management of persistent *unharmonious ARC* is to remove diplopia, by the least prism strength possible, or surgery to restore the earlier squint angle, or by the methods of diplopia control described above (see 4.3). Usually, unharmonious ARC is transient.

4.8   Classification of amblyopia

Amblyopia is a unilateral or bilateral decrease of vision for which no obvious cause can be detected by the physical examination of the eye and which in appropriate cases is correctable by therapeutic measures.

The main causes are (i) abnormal binocular interaction, (ii) foveal form vision deprivation and (iii) a combination of (i) and (ii).

Organic types of amblyopia

1   Organic amblyopia, due to disease: e.g. Stargardt's juvenile macular dystrophy, macular haemorrhage due to birth trauma, demyelinating neuropathy.

2   Congenital amblyopia, a developmental anomaly also known as cone deficiency syndrome which is bilateral and in its full form shows nystagmus, poor colour vision, and poor acuity. It also presents as a partial form.

3   Toxic amblyopia, due to lead, methanol, chloroquine, steroids, tobacco.

4   Hysterical amblyopia: conversion arising from anxiety, depression, and/or phobias.

Functional types of amblyopia

1 Refractive types of amblyopia (synonym: ametropic amblyopia)
   (i)   bilateral high hypermetropia, astigmatism; myopia (partially organic)
   (ii) anisometropia, over two dioptres spherical or astigmatic error
  (iii) meridional amblyopia.
2 Stimulus deprivation amblyopia, due to opacities, ptosis.
3 Nystagmus induced amblyopia (may be partially organic).
4 Strabismic amblyopia, (synonym: suppression amblyopia) including microstrabismus.

4.9 Obsolete terminology

The obsolete terms *amblyopia of arrest* and *amblyopia of extinction* refer to Chavasse's theory that the level of amblyopia related to the age of onset (Chavasse, 1939). Visual acuity is now known to develop faster than Chavasse believed and also to be capable of improvement later. Amblyopia depth is related more to the length of time that an eye is strabismic rather than the age of onset. The even older term *amblyopia of disuse* (amblyopia ex anopsia) is difficult to sustain following the discovery of active suppression mechanisms and the active adaptation of ARC.

The terms 'morphoscopic' for linear acuity, and 'angular' for single letter acuity are not appropriate.

4.10 Prevalence and characteristics of amblyopia

The prevalence of amblyopia in the general population is about 2.5%, but of course higher in ophthalmic practice. In 6-year-old children the overall incidence is 4%; in those with accommodative and partially accommodative squint it is 21% and in those with non-accommodative squint it is 35%. Amblyopia is less common in exotropes, many of whom are intermittent, and those hypermetropes who may have some binocular control in certain directions of gaze (von Noorden, 1985).

In strabismic amblyopia the visual acuity does not reduce uniformly as the image is moved peripherally away from the fovea. Instead, there is a central zone of reduced acuity due to obligatory suppression. This is an active inhibition of acuity both cortically and through efferent neurones back to the retina. The effect is to produce a crater-like depression in the centre of the 'mountain' of visual acuity plotted across the retina. The best acuity is found on the rim of the crater where rods and cones are present. A 2.0 ND log unit filter will not reduce acuity since the presence of rods allows good mesopic acuity. The normal eye has a drop of one line on the Snellen chart from 6/5 to 6/9 per $\frac{1}{2}°$ (1^{Δ}) off the fovea, and then 1½° (3^{Δ}) per line. Organic amblyopes use the remnants of central acuity and they suffer a drop in acuity with a neutral density filter.

4.11   Investigation of amblyopia

Acuity may be tested from birth monocularly (and binocularly) with the Teller Acuity Cards or the Keeler Acuity Card System. The Catford nystagmus drum, Stycar rolling balls (Sheridan, 1969) and location of the tiny sweets called 'hundreds and thousands' (these are spherical and coloured, about 1 mm in diameter) are useful for comparing one eye with another but lack scientific validation, except for the Catford drum, which has been shown to be inaccurate. The Kay test (Kay Pictures, P.O. Box 156, Coventry, CV8 3LJ, UK) and the Sheridan Gardiner test can be used from 2 to 3 years old. Linear versions should be used in addition to single letter testing. A one-line difference in single letter testing as opposed to linear acuity can occur in normal children. But this would be in both eyes. More than this would indicate bilateral amblyopia. In an amblyopic eye, the difference between linear and single letter visual acuity may represent the improvement possible by treatment. In gross amblyopia, this may be an over-optimistic prognosis. The difference is called the **crowding phenomenon**.

When there is no difference between single letter and linear acuity, then the development of vision may have been completed. If this level is below normal an organic amblyopia may be present.

The Snellen chart is used as a standard visual acuity test. However it is good practice to monitor amblyopia by using more than one VA test (and also by using more than one stereopsis test). A Landolt broken circle chart is more precise. Logmar charts (such as the Ferris-Bailey) are used for research purposes, and ideally would be used for amblyopia monitoring. Contrast sensitivity tests have two variables: spatial frequency (like a Snellen chart) and contrast threshold. The stimuli are sine-wave gratings. Strabismic and anisometropic amblyopia show a characteristic loss (raised threshold) for high spatial frequency contrast sensitivity. Organic amblyopia shows a loss of medium and lower frequencies. The Arden grating book (American Optical Co.) is a clinical contrast sensitivity test and can be used to monitor amblyopia treatment (see 5.5).

Visual evoked cortical potentials can be used to assess acuity particularly in young children with multiple defects and older brain-damaged children (Apkarian *et al.*, 1981).

4.12   Eccentric fixation

Eccentric fixation hardly occurs under non-clinical conditions, except for 'micro-tropia with identity' (see 7.13). It is a monocular adaptation, and amblyopic patients fixate with the non-amblyopic eye. For the purposes of professional qualifying examinations and also for treatment, the features of eccentric fixation need to be known. Monocular fixation may be classified as follows:

1 Central: steady or unsteady.
2 Eccentric: steady or unsteady.
3 No fixation pattern evident.

The concept of *localization* presents difficulties. *Absolute localization* refers to the patient's interpretation from visual and proprioceptive information (e.g. from eye muscle contraction) of his position in space (Fig. 4.9). *Relative localization* refers to the localization of visual objects with reference to each eye separately. A recently paretic patient will get incorrect proprioceptive information and will *past point* (absolute). The diplopic images are correctly localized from each eye. However, a long-standing squinter with anomalous retinal correspondence will not past point (absolute) but will localize the position of visual objects from one eye incorrectly (relative), e.g. a Bagolini streak, under binocular conditions.

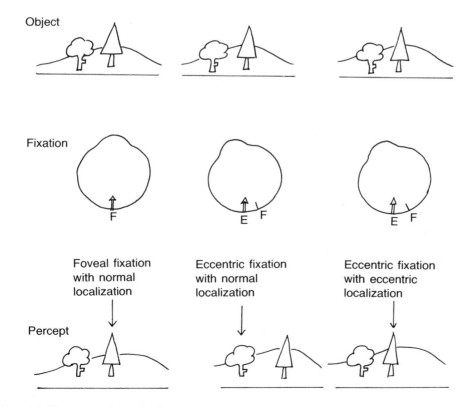

Fig. 4.9 Fixation and localization.

In eccentric fixation the relative localization may be as follows:

1   At the eccentrically fixating retinal point, relative localization may be normal or abnormal.
2   At the fovea of the same eye, relative localization may be normal or abnormal.

If the fovea has lost normal (central) localization, the prognosis for amblyopia treatment is poor. The fixation reflex has been referred to the eccentrically fixating retinal point.

In microtropia, it is common to find that the angles of the deviation, of the (ARC) anomaly, and of the monocular eccentric fixation are identical: *microtropia with identity*, (see 7.13).

The diagnosis of eccentric fixation is generally made using an ophthalmoscope. The patient is asked to look at the eccentric fixation graticule (see Fig. 4.10). If the patient does fixate the graticule with the fovea there will be no foveal reflex since the graticule is black. If eccentric fixation is present the foveal reflex may still be occluded by part of the graticule, or else it will be dimmed by the green filter. Ophthalmoscopes such as the Visuscope 2000 can have test chart graticules which allow assessment of monocular fixation facility both objectively and subjectively. In general however, it may be better to use the macular stop of an ophthalmoscope, first calibrating its size by projecting it on the optic disc, which subtends 5° by 7° (8^Δ by 12^Δ). The patient should then be asked to fixate the centre of the aperture and then the top, bottom, right and left edges to assess fixation. Eccentric fixation should be recorded, e.g. '2 degrees nasal, steady'. Loss of foveal localization may be checked by placing the macular stop or a graticule on the fovea and inquiring whether it appears straight ahead or to one side. If it is seen to one side then foveal localization is no longer central.

Fig. 4.10 Eccentric fixation graticules.

Other tests for eccentric fixation include

1   Amsler chart: the position of distortion or a gap in the grid will indicate the degree of eccentricity. The Threshold Amsler Grid (Stereo Optical Co, Chicago, Illinois 60641, USA) which uses contra-rotating polarized filters for each eye allows a more sensitive test for the scotoma.

2   Corneal reflection: following measurement of angle lambda in the better eye, any difference in this angle in the amblyopic eye may be due to eccentric fixation, assuming the angle lambda is equal for each eye.

3   Past pointing: the patient's better eye is occluded. The patient then points at a fixation target within arms reach. Past pointing indicates eccentric fixation with abnormal localization.

4   Blind spot plotting: if the amblyopic blind spot is at a different angle to that of the better eye, the degree of eccentricity can be measured.

5   Boer and Hofstetter's 'Purkinje tree' method: a pinhole is moved circularly to produce a tree effect.

4.13   Management of amblyopia

Organic types of amblyopia will need medical treatment of the underlying disease, toxicity or psychosomatic disorder. Functional types of amblyopia will need refractive and iseikonic correction, treatment of any ptosis or opacity where practicable, occlusion and active amblyopia therapy. In some cases prisms or drugs can be used. A full ophthalmic examination including ophthalmoscopy, visual fields, motility and pupil reflexes should be given before treatment is undertaken.

Passive therapy: refractive correction and occlusion

For babies up to 1 year, whose amblyopia exceeds the Teller Acuity Card norms (see Table 1.1), give occlusion of the better eye for one quarter of the baby's waking hours for straight-eyed amblyopia; but in strabismus, for half the waking hours. Review in 2 weeks. Gross refractive errors (over 4 dioptres spherical, 2 dioptres astigmatism or 2 dioptres anisometropia) would ideally be corrected by extended wear contact lenses, or failing that, miotics, and failing that by miosis achieved by a reasonable illumination level.

Between 1 and 2 years, the good eye would be patched for half the child's waking hours. Occlusion should be accompanied by some visual stimulation such as looking at moving coloured lights or pictures. A game of 'Peep-Bo' is likely to attract the child's interest, i.e. hiding and re-presenting interesting toys and dolls. Binocular stimulation with a black and white chequered light box for brief periods may help to improve acuity and reduce suppression. This is shown in diagrammatic form in Fig. 4.11 (see Reinecke, 1978). Ideally, regular assessment of visual acuity should be made with the Teller or Keeler Acuity Cards. This avoids the risk of inducing stimulus-deprivation amblyopia in the occluded eye. *The damage to binocularly driven cortical neurones is now thought to be a consequence of strabismus, and not occlusion* (von Noorden, 1985).

By 3 to 4 years old, several hours daily total occlusion of the better eye may be prescribed using non-allergenic Opticlude occluders. The occluder should

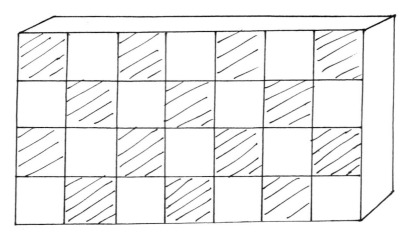

Fig. 4.11 The chequer-board light box (diagrammatic).

be removed at intervals to avoid stimulus deprivation amblyopia (occlusion amblyopia) in the 'good' eye. This should be done every third day in children in their third year, and every fourth day in the fourth year. There is no need to transfer occlusion to the other eye if acuities are monitored monthly, because the occurrence of stimulus deprivation amblyopia can be detected immediately and remedied. Mere removal of the occluder will give the fixating eye all the stimulus necessary.

Where occlusion causes distress in children under 4 years, it may be possible to occlude for shorter daily periods. This will be better than nothing. Constant occlusion should be the aim from 4 years on, where a squint is present. If the eyes are straight, part-time occlusion or constant partial occlusion (e.g. Fablon) may be given for a compliant child who will look through his glasses and not over the top. It is important to obtain the maximum improvement before the child goes to school.

Occlusion amblyopia (i.e. of the good eye) is reversible. The appearance of occlusion amblyopia does indicate a good prognosis for the amblyopic eye. Occlusion also helps to prevent the development or reinforcement of anomalous retinal correspondence in a pre-school child. In a patient with a marked hetero-phoria, occlusion may produce an intermittent tropia, with diplopia. *Prolonged occlusion in a child over 8 years with a deep harmonious ARC may increase the squint angle, and may thus produce diplopia.* The parents should be aware of this possibility. The remedy is to monitor the patient at 1- or 2-monthly intervals, where this risk exists.

Results may be obtained quickly in young children, with improvement as fast as one Snellen line a fortnight. Even a 6/60 acuity may rapidly improve. However, from 4 or 5 years old, a 6/60 acuity coupled with marked anisometropia may take 3 months to improve to 6/36 and so on. If there is no improvement after 3–6 months, treatment may be discontinued. In these cases visual field measurements should be repeated to rule out the gradual development of any disease which could produce organic amblyopia. From 4 years old, children can usually co-operate with a multiple stimulus screener such as the Henson or Friedmann. Under this age a careful ophthalmoscopic check for tilted discs or other disc abnormalities can be made, and the swinging flashlight (pupil reflex) test performed for unilateral organic amblyopia. When the acuity has stabilised, treatment should be withdrawn gradually as there is a risk that the amblyopia may recur. For example, occlusion should be dropped from constant to one hour daily for a month, and the VA checked then, and again after a further month, without occlusion. Illness may produce a marked increase in an apparently stable amblyopia in a pre-teenage child, probably due to increased suppression consequent to binocular instability. Management of any deviation should be undertaken at the same time as the amblyopia treatment.

Amblyopia in unilateral high myopia has a 25% chance of improvement when picked up on entering school and a decision may be taken with the parents on whether or not to treat (von Noorden, 1985). Similarly, in anisometropic amblyopia of 6/36 or so in a 10- to 12-year-old, treatment may be inappropriate. In these cases it is important not only to record the decision but also the discussion with the parents. When the child is trying to get a job at the age of 17 in an occupation requiring good vision there may well be a feeling that treatment should have been given. One way around this problem is to give treatment for 3 months when the child is first seen, and then confirm with the parents the decision to discontinue therapy.

For children presenting with amblyopia at school entry, the teacher should be informed about the need for constant occlusion. This should be given at least for 2 months. In individual cases where the child is distressed by physical occlusion (e.g. in asthmatic children if the distress precipitates asthma), atropine (mainly in hospital practice) or cyclopentolate occlusion may be prescribed. After the initial 2 months it may be necessary to go to part-time occlusion. This should cover all non-school hours and include specific exercises for a total of 20–30 minutes daily.

In eccentric fixation with eccentric localization (see 4.12) direct occlusion of the fixing eye is contra-indicated, as there is a risk of encouraging the eccentric localization. Instead, pleoptic techniques would be used.

Active therapy: exercises

Home exercises include:

1 For infants, a chequer-board light box which flashes to provide visual stimulation has been described (see Awaya, 1978). In addition to treating amblyopia, this reduces binocular adaptations such as suppression and anomalous correspondence. This is because even in the presence of a squint, adjacent black and white squares can be fused (see Fig. 4.11). (To understand this, hold your hands in front of you, palm to palm, and with the back of one hand towards your face. Now slide your hands sideways apart, by one digit. You can still 'fuse' the two hands.)

2 Small writing in coloured ink.

3 Dotting: the child fills a series of circles drawn around a coin with dots, counts them and numbers the circle.

4 Crossing out the letters 'e' and 'o' in a newspaper.

5 Red filter treatment: the amblyopic eye is occluded except for exercise periods of 1–3 hours daily when the occluder is swapped, and a Lee Primary Red 106 or Lee Light Red 182 red filter attached to the spectacle lens of the amblyopic eye. These filters have a 50% transmittance at 620 and 650 nm respectively (Lee Filters, Central Way, Walworth, Andover, Hants., UK).

6 The CAM stimulator (Campbell *et al.*, 1978) treats amblyopia by rotating gratings, but has been the subject of some criticism (Douthwaite *et al.*, 1981).

7 The Mallett Intermittent Photic Stimulator Unit (IPS) combines red light stimulation at 4 Hz with an interesting and detailed visual task, for 20–30 minutes once or twice a week. The task detail must be recognized, counted and traced where possible.

8 A variety of pleoptic techniques have been described (Bangerter, 1950; Cüppers, 1956). These were particularly useful for neglected amblyopia. Later, the Keeler Projectoscope with the Nutt Autodisc was developed. This ophthalmoscope allows the location of a marker target onto the amblyopic fovea. A brilliant flash then dazzles the surrounding area, leaving only the fovea without an after-image. The instrument then delivers a gently pulsating light and graticule stimulus. This is effective, but needs an (alternate day) 10-minute session for 2 weeks to get a typical improvement of one Snellen line. Other forms of therapy should be given concurrently to maintain the improvement.

9 For older schoolchildren (over 8 years old) 'after-image transfer' can be used (Caloroso, 1972). A small 5 mm square black occluder is placed in the centre of a photographic flashgun. The flashgun is held in front of the better eye at such a distance that the black square subtends the angle of the smallest letter recognized with the amblyopic eye. The amblyopic eye is occluded and the flash is discharged. A suitable ultra-violet light filter should cover the flash aperture (see Charman, 1989). A suitable filter can be obtained from Lee Filters (see 5 above). The occluder is swapped to the better eye and the after-image is projected, as if by the fovea of the amblyopic eye, as a light coloured square. The patient reads

down the Snellen chart, placing the after-image on each letter in turn thus utilizing the amblyopic fovea rather than the eccentric areas either side which might have better acuity. The after-image can be replenished by switching the room lights off and on occasionally, for at least 5 minutes. This technique requires a co-operative patient. It is contra-indicated in ARC over 1.5 ND units, and for anisometropic amblyopia.

10 'Inverse prism' treatment combines constant full occlusion of the good eye with a 6^Δ to 20^Δ base-out prism for temporal eccentric fixation (base-in for nasal). This requires a re-learning of the correct monocular hand–eye co-ordination. The prism strength is given to marginally exceed the angle of eccentric fixation.

11 Amblyopia and oculomotor deviations are normally treated simultaneously. Physiological diplopia exercises may be used in squint angles under 12^Δ, with an initial VA of 6/24 or better, (see 6.11, 6.12 and Pickwell, 1989).

12 'Penalisation' originally referred to therapeutic occlusion using cycloplegia, but is also used to describe partial occlusion by refractive fogging. It is accompanied by active therapy.

CHAPTER 5
Clinical Investigation of Binocular Anomalies

5.1   History checklist

1   Family history of ocular deviations and visual disability including cousins, uncles, aunts, grandparents, and children and their treatment.

2   Pre-natal and delivery problems. Was the mother an in-patient before delivery, ask about unplanned caesarian section, forceps (Fig. 5.1) or breech delivery, fetal distress, was the child kept in hospital more than 3 days, did the paediatrician make any comment, was delivery pre-term (earlier than 32 weeks), was there low or very low birth weight, was oxygen needed, was there retinopathy of prematurity?

3   Developmental problems, illness — especially pyrexia or fits, separation from parents, hyper- or hypo-activity, any medication, accidental or non-accidental head injury, crossed hand and eye dominance?

4   Age and mode (sudden or gradual) of onset — usually intermittent, when tired or ill. A sudden onset may indicate a more serious cause.

5   Was the onset associated with any other factor? Educational problems: general or specific e.g. dyslexia and associated language problems, mirror writing, comprehension difficulty. Health problems: systemic disease, diabetes, thyroid, inborn errors of metabolism, skeletal dysgenesis, facial asymmetry, hearing deficit.

6   Has the direction of the deviation changed spontaneously or following treatment?

7   Was there an abnormal head posture — any photographs — head turn and/or tilt may be towards affected muscle to reduce the need to rely on it, or to the opposite direction to widen diplopic images and reduce confusion.

8   What was the delay between first onset and first treatment? When were glasses, occlusion exercises or surgery given?

5.2   Associated ocular abnormalities

Pupil size, equality and reflexes; monocular accommodation, ptosis, heterochromia iridis (? uveitis, mesodermal dysgenesis), blepharospasm, myokymia

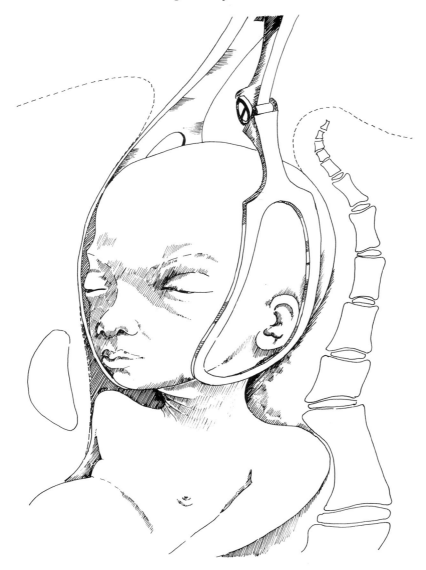

Fig. 5.1 Forceps delivery. Note that the forceps are more likely to produce raised intra-cranial pressure than localized trauma.

(fatigue), nystagmus (type). Head tilt or turn or chin depression/elevation (as in A or V patterns).

5.3 Symptoms

Few symptoms may be reported by the child. Rather, signs may be noticed by parent, grandparent or health visitor or there may be failure of a pre-school, school or occupational vision test. However, possible symptoms include *blurred vision* — maybe intermittently. This could be a description of confusion and diplopia. Alternatively the patient may be accommodating and sacrificing clear vision in order to avoid diplopia. When patients see double they sometimes complain of 'everything going into one'. Exophoria may decompensate in high illumination levels, say 5000 lux or above. The patient typically will close one eye. If *diplopia* is present then check: is it physiological or pathological, momentary or prolonged, in the direction of paresis only, for distance and/or for near vision, triplopia, monocular diplopia, effect of glasses e.g. new anisometropic Rx, bifocals badly fitted or loose?

Vertigo may be associated with oculogyric crisis (see 9.11) or a vestibular lesion, or associated with nausea and headaches: a possible intracranial space occupying lesion. Oculogyric eye rolling may occur with pyrexia and in brain-damaged children. It may also be learned.

Headaches: where? how long? how often? how bad? associated with sinusitis, occupation, time of day.

Pain on eye movement may be associated with a restrictive paresis.

Other symptoms including closing or covering of one eye, falling over or bumping into things, tactile difficulty, difficulty with playing ball games, parking a car, threading a needle, or pegging washing on a clothes line. In A and V pattern incomitancy a head up or down position may be adopted to maintain binocularity.

5.4 Refraction and current correction

The refraction, cycloplegic and post-cycloplegic refraction should be noted, together with the current correction. In particular any under or over-correction should be recorded.

In the Professional Qualifying Examination (PQE) both the refraction and the correction including prisms, if any are given, and the correction should be assumed to be optimal. It is important to know whether the glasses include a fogging element in one lens and the full description of prism strength and base. Watch out for:

1 Bifocals prescribed for orthoptic reasons.
2 Negative lenses (or a reduced positive correction) prescribed for poor convergence, or for divergence excess.

The latter may exist either as a phoria, or as a tropia.

5.5   Vision and visual acuity (VA)

From birth until 2 years old vision may be measured by Teller Acuity Cards or by Keeler Acuity Cards. These tests include manuals giving the norms for babies and children from birth. From post-term age in months (see Table 1.1) binocular VA is somewhat higher than monocular, but both show a range of normal values. Note the plateau around 8 to 12 months old, where VA does not improve. Normal acuity (6/5) is attained at 3 years on these tests. From 2 years, use Sheridan Gardiner tests using five, seven or nine letter symbols. The Sonksen Silver Acuity System (Keeler) is a useful development of the Sheridan Gardiner test. It has the added advantage of linear presentation of the optotypes, with standardized spacing. The Egan Calver test type works on similar principles. The Cambridge Crowding Cards (Clement Clarke International) have a central letter surrounded by four other letters, and are used to measure the ratio between linear and single letter acuity. The Kay test (see 4.11) uses symbols of common objects, which a 2- or 3-year-old child can name, and is standardized against Snellen acuity.

It is usual to record the single letter acuity at first but as soon as the child's attention span allows, check linear acuity. A difference between these is described as the crowding phenomenon (see von Noorden, 1985). Such a difference may however be found in children subsequently found to be normal, providing the difference between linear and single letter acuity was equal for each eye. A different degree of crowding between right and left eyes would indicate an abnormality, e.g. strabismic amblyopia. Single letter acuity may represent the potential for good vision which is not yet attained in an amblyopic eye.

The Sheridan Gardiner test chart is mirror reversible so that it can be used at 6 m or 3 m. Modern test cabinets often allow the chart to be removed easily and replaced, and a Sheridan Gardiner version is available.

The effect of a 2.0 ND filter (ND value = 1/log transmission) on visual acuity will demonstrate the better performance in mesopic conditions of strabismic and anisometropic amblyopia. In organic amblyopia VA drops markedly under these conditions.

Amsler chart testing may show a central area of reduced acuity in the amblyopic eye. Contrast sensitivity tests such as the American Optical Book based on Arden's work and the VisTech Consultants chart also will show reduced response to high-frequency stimuli in functional amblyopia. Other contrast sensitivity tests include the Pelli-Robson letter CS chart, the Cambridge low contrast gratings, and the Tunnacliffe low contrast letter chart. Progress in amblyopia treatment should be monitored both by high contrast (e.g. Snellen charts) and by contrast sensitivity.

Visual acuity in infants may be assessed by optokinetic nystagmus using variable width gratings projected on to a curved screen, and by visually evoked cortical potentials, sometimes called the visual evoked response (VER). The latter may also be modified to assess stereopsis.

5.6   Cover test: introduction

The *objective cover test* should be carried out at 6 m and at 33 cm on an accommodative target which is at, or slightly above, the acuity level of the more amblyopic eye. The cover test recovery speed should be noted as it indicates the degree of control over a decompensated phoria. The cover test should be repeated above and below the primary position to detect V and A patterns of incomitancy. The easiest way to arrange this is to get the patient to tilt the chin 15° or 20° up and then perform the cover test. Repeat with the chin tilted down.

The *habitual angle* is found by briefly covering the fixing eye and increasing the amount of prism in front of the deviating eye until any movement is neutralized. An error can occur with the prism cover test due to the deviated visual axis failing to pass through the optical centre of the correcting spectacle lens. A further error will be produced by incorrect centring or any prism in the lens.

The *total squint angle* is found by covering each eye alternately until no further cover test movement is seen. The difference between habitual and total angles may be marked in esotropia with an accommodative element. Both measurements are therefore necessary to decide the management.

The *subjective cover test* may be used to detect very small angles of squint (see 5.11). The patient looks at a spotlight and is asked to report any apparent movement of it when either eye is occluded − this would indicate a squint. It would only occur in the minority of microtropia cases which do not have 'microtropia with identity' (see 4.12 and 7.13). The subjective cover test may also be used as an initial guide to the habitual strabismus angle. Raise the prism bar in front of the deviating eye until diplopia is reported. The angle indicated just before diplopia occurs corresponds to the objective cover test. It is obtained very much more rapidly than with objective prism cover testing and is a useful preliminary technique, for example in the professional qualifying examination.

Cyclophoria may be assessed with red and white Maddox rods, placed one before each eye, which are rotated to provide a subjective impression of being vertical. For near fixation, a Maddox Wing test can be used.

5.7   Cover test technique

Initially it is important to check that the patient's head position is normal. A head tilt or turn may invalidate the result. Later the head may be moved to look for an A or V pattern. To begin the cover test (strictly, the *cover–uncover test*), the patient should keep his glasses on if they are normally worn for distance vision.

The patient is asked to look at an accommodative target such as a 6/9 letter if both eyes have normal VA – it is difficult to concentrate on a letter at the limit of resolution. Where accommodation is likely to be affecting the squint angle, the patient should be asked to read out the whole line of letters immediately before fixating one letter and having the cover test performed. In amblyopia, choose a letter which can just be seen by the amblyopic eye. Use a spotlight if you can be certain that there is no active accommodation, or if the amblyopic acuity is below 6/18, or for subjective cover testing. Both the general illumination (2000 lux) and the local illumination on the patient's face should be at a high level, but without producing discomfort or disability glare, which could produce decompensation of a phoria or an increase in the angle of a tropia.

The test distances are 20 m for detection of intermittent exotropia, 6 m and 33 cm for routine testing and 15 cm for suspected convergence excess tropia, particularly in infants with short spans of attention. For near fixation use an accommodative target on a fixation stick.

First, fully cover the eye you suspect to be normally fixing for about 1 second: count 'one little second'. The white side of the occluder should be towards the patient's eye in order to maximize the illumination on the eye. Watch the other eye for any movement to take up fixation. In deep amblyopia (<6/36) there may be a delay, so ask the patient whether he or she is looking straight at the fixation target. Consider the possibility of eccentric fixation. If eccentric fixation is found later on in the examination, the amount of eccentricity in prism dioptres must be *added* to the prism cover test result. This is assuming the eccentricity is nasal and the patient is esotropic or temporal in exotropia.

Next, observe the eye behind the cover by placing yourself in the monocular (temporal) field of that eye and looking behind the cover. Do not allow the patient to use his binocular visual field. Remove the cover vertically so that you do not cover test yourself inadvertently. Watch for any movement of the previously covered eye to regain fixation. Note the speed of recovery as this is a guide to compensation in heterophoria. A rapid recovery indicates a compensated phoria. A double movement of regress (recovery) may be seen. This is believed to indicate first a tropia-induced deviation and then a 'phoria' which may occur in patients with unstable anomalous retinal correspondence. Another explanation may be that the double movement is caused by the total and habitual elements of the squint.

If no cover test movement is seen with the cover–uncover test, apply the *alternate cover test*. Cover each eye in turn, finally leaving the occluder covering the eye with the better acuity. Remove and then re-apply the occluder to see whether a small angle tropia can now be detected.

Repeat the cover test on the other eye. Avoid being psychologically set for horizontal eye movements only. A small lid movement may accompany vertical deviations. Vertical deviations may become more apparent following surgery for horizontal heterotropia. Oblique deviations are conventionally recorded as a combination of the vertical and horizontal elements; only one deviation is present of course. Oblique deviations may be measured by a prism cover test in the direction of the smaller element (vertical or horizontal) first. A single correcting prism of that amount is then placed in the trial frame, and the other element is measured with an appropriate prism bar (Fig. 5.2), vertical or horizontal type as appropriate. An alternative technique is to use a single prism bar held obliquely, so as to neutralize the oblique deviation with a single measurement. In this case the base of the measuring prism should be recorded, using a 360° notation, as well as the prism strength.

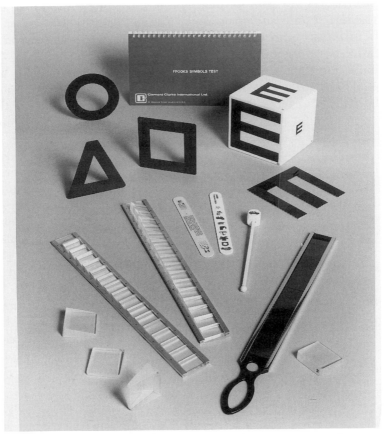

Fig. 5.2 Orthoptic equipment: vertical and horizontal prism bars, loose prisms, the Bagolini red filter bar, fixation ('budgie') sticks, the Lang fixation cube (there is a picture on each face, and one on the end), the Ffookes and 'E' acuity tests.

If no eye movement has been found by cover test so far, *alternate* the occluder between each eye several times, finally holding it over one eye. Remove the occluder and look for any phoria movement of recovery. Repeat, leaving the occluder over the other eye. If still no cover test movement has been seen, repeat the cover test leaving the occluder over each eye for 3 seconds instead of 1 second before removal: this will demonstrate quite marked exophoria, up to 10^Δ to 20^Δ in some patients.

If so far the patient appears orthophoric, apply the *subjective cover test*. This test utilizes one aspect of the 'phi phenomenon'. The patient looks at a spotlight at 6 m, and the unilateral and alternate cover test are performed asking the patient to report any jump or change in position of the spotlight. Many 'straight eyed' anisometropic amblyopes could also be classified as microtropias. Placing a Bagolini lens in front of such an eye will occasionally reveal the Bagolini streak to one side of the spotlight. This is a small angle squint with normally suppressed NRC or unharmonious ARC. This particular small angle squint therefore does not come strictly within the current classification of microtropia.

During routine orthoptic assessment it is often appropriate to complete motility and sensory status tests with the patient continuing to wear the refractive correction. This avoids the disadvantages of unwanted changes in the binocular motor and sensory status, such as a phoria becoming decompensated. Having completed these tests, you should then return to the cover test, this time without the refractive correction, in order to assess the effect of the refractive correction on the binocular motor status.

5.8   Estimation of deviation angle

The current P.Q.E. Syllabus and Guidelines require a candidate either to estimate or measure the angle of strabismus. Measurement, particularly by prism cover test, will give an accurate measurement of the total squint angle. Estimation has the advantage of giving the habitual angle of strabismus, but can be quite inaccurate when used by a novice.

1 The practitioner can practise estimation of the angle of the deviation on a subject who shifts binocular fixation 2, 4, 6 (etc.) prism dioptres on a tangent screen.

2 Ask the patient to look from one end to the other of a 6/9 line — if 12 cm in width at 6 m this is a 2 prism dioptre movement. Repeat with 4 and 6 prism dioptre movements using appropriately wider targets on the test chart or in the room. Next perform the cover test and compare the cover test movement to the previous binocular version movement, or multiples of it.

3 Estimations of squint angles are traditionally made in degrees, measurements in prism dioptres (except cyclophoria). However, it is good practice to record all deviations in prism dioptres — avoid degrees — and indicate whether measured or estimated e.g. 'CT $20^\triangle$ R SOT (estimated)'. For small angles, $4° = 7^\triangle$, (and so $11° = 20^\triangle$ and $22° = 40^\triangle$).

4 The Hirschberg corneal reflection test estimates 1 mm of decentration of the corneal reflex as $7°$ ($12^\triangle$) deviation which gives $25°$ for a reflex on the pupil edge and $45°$ on the limbus.

5 The more precise Krimsky prism reflex test requires the patient to fixate a penlight and prisms are increased in front of the *fixing eye* (not the deviating eye as in the cover test) until the corneal reflex in the deviated eye is centred.

6 For greater accuracy the *angle lambda* (often called 'angle kappa' which is technically incorrect) should be measured first (see Fig. 5.3). The patient looks at one end of a 15 cm ruler while a pen torch is moved along the ruler until its corneal reflection is in the centre of the pupil. If the ruler is 50 cm from the patient's eye, the distance along the ruler in centimetres multiplied by two gives the angle lambda in prism dioptres. Repeat for the other eye.

7 If the corneal reflexes are central or symmetrical in both eyes and there is no other indication of a squint, the Hirschberg result should be recorded in addition to the cover test, in the case of children under 3 years, as additional evidence of normal binocular function.

8 The angle of a deviation may be precisely (but not accurately) measured with a haploscope, such as a synoptophore, or single mirror haploscope. These

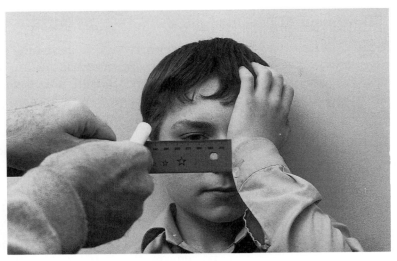

Fig. 5.3 Angle lambda measurement. The patient fixates one end of a ruler, held 50 cm away. The pen torch is moved along the ruler until the corneal reflex is seen in the centre of the pupil. The distance in cm. multiplied by two, gives angle lambda in prism dioptres.

instruments provide a useful assessment of changes in motor and sensory status over a period of time. They are also useful for therapy. But they are less reliable for absolute measurements. They suffer from proximal convergence, and synotype instruments have only a 20° field of view, with greatly reduced illumination. For pre-operative assessment, a prism cover test is preferable. The synoptophore measurements are made by switching off the right and left illuminated (small circle and square) targets in turn and moving the arms of the instrument until no eye movement occurs — the objective angle. The patient then moves one arm of the synoptophore until the images overlap — the subjective angle. The difference is referred to as the *angle of the anomaly*. The single mirror haploscope measurement is made by the examiner performing a cover test and rotating the mirror until any eye movement stops.

9 Although the *Marlow prolonged occlusion test* is rarely used deliberately now, incidental occlusion of one eye for 1–14 days may well produce some surprising results, such as a large, compensated vertical phoria or horizontal deviation. Such occlusion may occur where one eye is bandaged or suffers a temporary reduction in vision for some reason.

10 In heterophoria, the Maddox rod and wing should be used in addition to the cover test. A *flip prism* of 1^Δ strength may be used superimposed on a Maddox rod (and mounted on a crossed cylinder flipper) to establish orthophoria by flipping the red streak either side, and then above and below, the 6 m fixation light (see 6.4).

5.9 Prism cover test measurement: further details

The patient should fixate a target at 6 m — a letter equal to (or, in the author's opinion, one line above) the amblyopic eye's acuity is the first choice. In patients with limited attention or with any accommodative element fully corrected, a spotlight may be used. (In the P.Q.E. the accommodative status may not be known, and a letter will be the best option). A prism bar is placed in front of the deviated eye with its plane surface next to the eye and the fixing eye is occluded. (Note that prescription lenses incorporating prisms have the prism worked on the surface next to the eye. This may make a difference to the effective strength in the higher powers.)

The prism is increased until the deviated eye ceases to make a movement to take up fixation when the other eye is covered. Do not stack prisms with their bases in the same direction unless you have a computer program to work out the additive effect. For example, $40^\Delta + 5^\Delta = 58^\Delta$; $40^\Delta + 10^\Delta = 100^\Delta$. For the near prism cover test, the prism must be held close to the eye — a 40^Δ exotropia at near fixation will measure 48^Δ if the prism is held 5 cm from the eye. Different base directions do not produce an additive error. If you do not have a strong enough prism, it is slightly better to split the prisms between the eyes.

A rapid initial guide to the angle of deviation may be obtained by sliding the prism bar to increase the prism until diplopia is reported on a spotlight. The retinal image of the spotlight will move from the fixation point to the fovea in the deviated eye and this area may show suppression under these conditions. Once past the fovea there will be no suppression and the light will be seen double. At this point the prism may be increased and decreased to find the objective measurement of squint angle.

Where a deviation is oblique it is possible to hold a vertical or horizontal prism bar obliquely and record the amount of the deviation in prism dioptres, and the base of the prism bar in degrees on a 360° protractor basis: extending the 0−180° protractor used for cylindrical axis recording. Alternatively the smaller of the vertical and horizontal components of an oblique deviation can be corrected with loose prisms in the trial frame and the larger components measured with the appropriate prism bar. If both components are large get the patient to hold one prism bar once one component has been measured and move the other prism bar to measure the other component.

Having made a rapid estimation of the squint angle by pushing up the prism bar until diplopia is reported, briefly occlude the fixing eye to establish the *habitual squint angle*. Then alternately cover each eye and increase the prism strength until no further eye movement occurs: this is the amount of the *total squint angle*.

5.10   Motility

Reflex motility tests the smooth pursuit eye movement system including the ocular motor nerves and muscles. The test can be performed objectively by watching any under- or over-action of eye movement in each diagnostic direction of gaze (see Fig. 5.4). If a non-focussed spotlight torch is used as the fixation target any (gross) relative change in corneal reflection between the two eyes may be seen. To do this the observer should theoretically move with the light source to avoid parallax. A subjective response can be obtained by asking whether the patient sees the light double in any direction, or whether it hurts, or is difficult to move the eyes in a specific direction of gaze. A focussed spotlight torch might easily be directed more towards one eye than the other. This would make observation of the reflex and the recognition of diplopia more difficult. The spotlight torch should be moved in a curve around the patient's head, as if on a perimeter arc, until the eyes stop moving. This will produce equal speeds and amounts of eye movement. It will avoid the error of performing the motility test over too small an area to detect all under and overactions. The Hess and Lees screens both have 'pincushion' distortion to correct for these tests being made on a plane surface. If a near fixation spatula (e.g. a 'budgie stick' from Clement

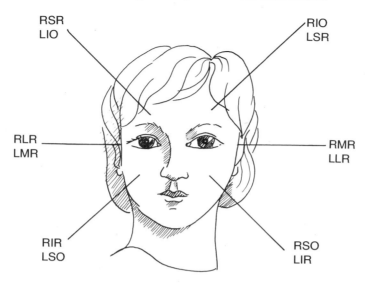

Fig. 5.4 Motility diagram: the cardinal diagnostic directions of gaze.

Clarke International) is used instead of the spotlight torch, diplopia will be seen as two fixation spatulas and any *torsional element* in the diplopia will be easily identified. One image of the spatula will appear tilted.

Where there is any doubt about the motility test result, it is useful to carry out a cover test in the diagnostic directions of gaze: the 'Union Jack' positions, except for the vertical line. A larger cover test movement in one direction will indicate an overaction by one eye and an underaction by the other eye, in that position.

If binocular motility is inconclusive, or where there is a very large squint angle which cannot be altered by correcting the refractive error, then monocular motility should be assessed without the refractive correction. If one eye is blind, it may be necessary to check its motility by asking the patient to look in each direction using voluntary control as the eye may drift off in binocular conditions and give a misleading result. Also check vertical motility movement for A or V patterns, and for lid lag which is a sign of hyperthyroidism.

The *advantages* of doing the motility test *with* the refractive correction in place is that if a squint has a large accommodative element, the angle might otherwise vary with the amount of accommodation, and an under- or over-action may appear to be present due to the large angle deviation.

The *advantages* of the motility test performed *without* spectacles are:

1   A small limitation of eye movement in a peripheral position of gaze may be seen more easily.

2   Small vertical up-shoots and down-shoots may be seen more readily, caused by restrictive paresis.

3   A larger amount of elevation and depression is available, for the assessment of A and V patterns.

It is therefore advisable to assess motility originally with, and then without glasses in place.

The *'doll's head phenomenon'* is useful in paresis. Forced gentle rotation of the head from side-to-side or vertically will normally produce eye movement in the opposite direction, unless the fixation reflex is too strong to allow this. If the lesion is supra-nuclear (or inter-nuclear) the eyes will deviate fully in the direction of an apparent paresis: the paresis disappears. If the lesion is infra-nuclear the paretic restriction of movement is still present.

Voluntary motility can be assessed by asking the patient to look up, down, right and left. This checks the frontal lobe function of voluntary eye movement.

The Parks head tilt test for vertical paresis is described in Chapter 8.

5.11   Diplopia fields

The diplopia fields may be plotted to assess the degree and directions in which diplopia occurs in incomitant deviations. This allows an appreciation of the patients problems and a method of monitoring the improvement or deterioration of the incomitancy or paresis. It is possible to construct a *tangent screen* or scale on which the patient fixates a white light into each direction of gaze. A red filter is placed in front of one eye and the patient reports the position of the red image on the screen. The red filter is then placed before the other eye and the test repeated. In paresis the secondary deviation, with paretic eye fixating the white light, will be greater than the primary deviation. The tangent screen is marked in prism dioptres. The diplopic area can then be shaded in on a field chart.

In routine practice it is simpler to draw a 3 × 3 *diplopia matrix* to record the horizontal and vertical elements of the deviation in each diagnostic direction of gaze (see Fig. 5.5). A red Maddox rod is placed before one eye and the refractive correction is worn to provide clear images and remove any accommodative element of a deviation. Alternatively, these measurements may be made by prism cover test in each direction of gaze. In order to standardize the directions of gaze the patient looks at a pen torch held 1 m away. The pen torch is moved in each diagnostic direction until one eye or both stop moving. This provides a fixed reference point for taking the measurement. Loose prisms may be used to measure the vertical element and a prism bar for the horizontal element.

The vertical result is recorded above the horizontal result in each of the nine boxes of the matrix. A second matrix is completed with the Maddox rod in front of the other eye. The results may be invalidated by ARC which may be fixed or

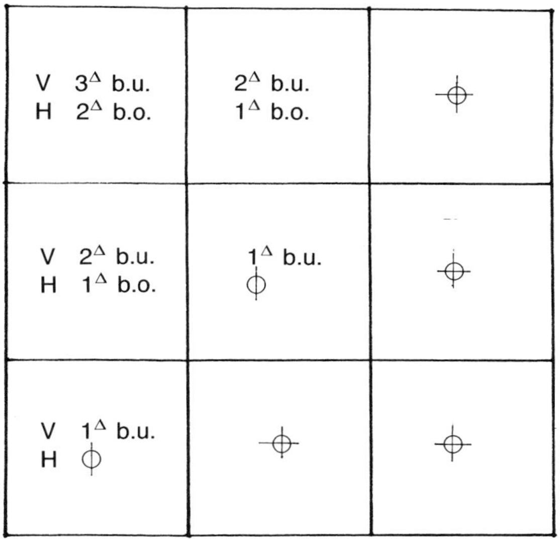

V 3^Δ b.u. H 2^Δ b.o.	2^Δ b.u. 1^Δ b.o.	$\oplus$
V 2^Δ b.u. H 1^Δ b.o.	1^Δ b.u. ϕ	$\oplus$
V 1^Δ b.u. H ϕ	$\oplus$	$\oplus$

Fig. 5.5 The diplopia matrix: b.u., base-up; b.o., base-out.

vary with the direction of gaze in old paresis. However, in practice, it is the progress of a recent paresis which needs monitoring, and here ARC will not occur.

The practical use of such a diplopia matrix is that it allows an estimation of the best compromise prism to prescribe, often in Fresnel form, to give maximum help to the patient over the whole binocular visual field.

5.12 Hess and Lee's screen tests

For the diagnosis of incomitancy and paresis a Hess screen is in common use. The original Hess screen utilized cords rather than projected images. A precursor, the Lancaster screen, used torches but did not have the curved plot required to correct for the tangential error introduced by recording eye rotations on a flat surface. The torches are known as Foster torches. The squares on the screen are at $5°$ (9^Δ) intervals, provided the patient sits $50\,cm$ from the screen.

The patient uses red and green goggles. Red and green TNO stereotest glasses may be used in most cases with greater convenience. The room illumination is reduced so that the patient only sees a red image with one eye and a green image with the other. Under these conditions any ARC may collapse and allow testing with NRC. It has been shown that in established paresis ARC may vary with the varying angle of deviation thus reducing or concealing incomitance. The red torch held by the examiner is projected onto the grey felt Hess screen

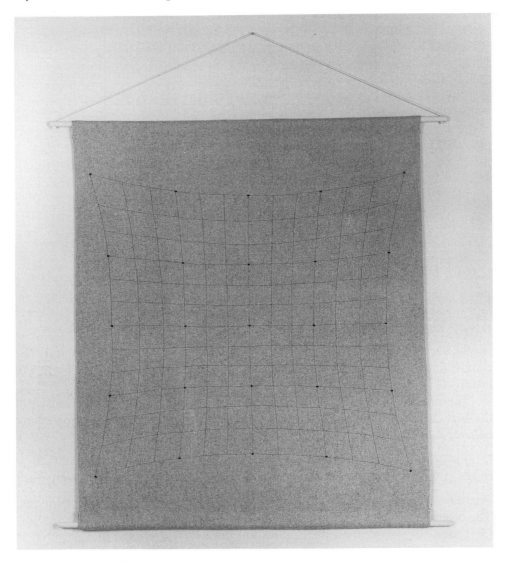

Fig. 5.6 The projection Hess screen.

(Fig. 5.6). The patient then projects his green torch to apparently superimpose the line images to make a cross. With children this can take the form of a space invaders game, the examiner's torch being switched off when the child's torch is aimed correctly. The new stimulus then appears at a different position on the Hess screen. After one eye has been plotted, the goggles are reversed. (In the case of TNO glasses, which can only be worn with the green glass in front of the right eye, the torches are swapped instead.) A uniform separation between the

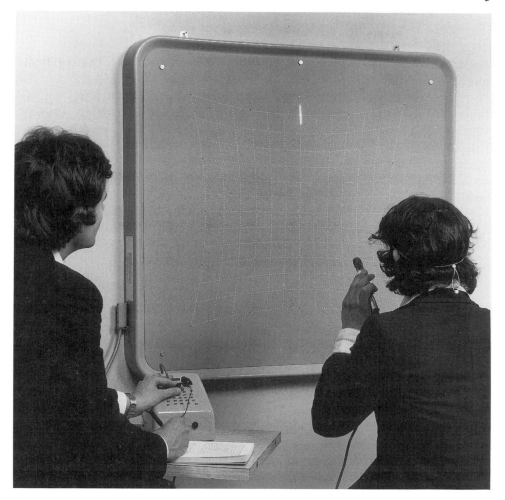

Fig. 5.7 The electric Hess screen.

red and green projected lines indicates a concomitant heterophoria or heterotropia. To interpret a Hess plot, the smaller area plot relates to the underacting eye. The most underacting muscle will be plotted furthest in restriction from the normal position. The contralateral synergist will be plotted furthest in overaction (see Figs. 8.1 to 8.8). Alternatively an electric Hess screen may be used (Fig. 5.6).

The Lee's screen is based on the Hess screen. The patient views one screen directly and another through a mirror. Only one screen is illuminated at a time. The patient points to each diagnostic point on the screen in turn. The examiner briefly switches the other screen on to record the result.

For examples of Hess screen charts, see Chapter 8. Figure 5.8 shows an

Fig. 5.8 Orthoptic record card.

FULL RECORD: ORTHOPTIC ASSESSMENT   Date:
Name   Occupation: Date of birth:
Address   Age:

Personal History: Birth: normal, unplanned caesarian, forceps, premature, oxygen.
Health visitor check (1 year):............Playgroup check ($3\frac{1}{2}$ years):.......
Hospital check: occlusion: surgery:
Last refractive correction: R..........L...........Add.....Date.........
Deviation onset: age:..........   Mode: intermittent, sudden........
Family history:....................   Heredity:..........................

Symptoms: *SUMMARY OF EYE PROBLEMS*
                               1.
                               2.
                               3.
                               4.

Refraction:
Non-cycloplegic: Vision:....   R........=V.A.: Vision:...   L.....=V.A
Cycloplegic Drug:.........   R......................   L..........
Eye disease/abnormality: Pupils: Lids: Media: Fundi: Fields:
Facial dissymmetry: Syndromes:
Binocular motor status: *By estimation with Rx*   *By $^\Delta$ cover test with Rx*
Cover test at 6 m:
Cover test at 33 cm:

                 By estimation without Rx   *By $^\Delta$ cover test without Rx*
Cover test at 6 m:
Cover test at 33 cm:

                 By estimation   *By $^\Delta$ cover test*
                 (Rx + Add +3)   *(Rx + Add +3)*
Cover test at 33 cm:

Therefore non-accom. element = $^\Delta$,   accom. = $^\Delta$,   convergence
excess = $^\Delta$
Speed of recovery in heterophoria with Rx at 6 m: at 33 cm:
Speed of recovery in heterophoria without Rx at 6 m: at 33 cm:
Maddox rod at 6 m (phoria) with Rx: Maddox Wing:
Gradient test....: Maddox Wing with +1.00 added: −1.00 added:
Tropia 6 m: Prism cover test   ..   ..   :   ..   ..   :
Therefore AC/A ratio =
Fixation disparity (associated phoria) at 6 m: at 33 cm:

Relative vergences at 6 m: Abduct: blur, break, recovery. Adduct: blur, break, recovery

Relative vergences at 33 cm:

Motility: Binocular with Rx   Monocular without Rx   R   L
            Binocular without Rx

Hess plot (attached): diagnosis = ...(Recent/old).

Tonometry in direction of underacting muscle: R . . . . L . . . . Non-/Restrictive.

Convergence: Push-up: Jump: Fatigue?:   Prism:
   Voluntary convergence possible?:   Good controlled divergence from NPC?:

Four (or greater) prism dioptre test:

Binocular sensory status:

Stereotest: Lang: TNO: Randot: Other:

Correspondence: NRC/HARC/HARC by Bag./Mallett test/synop/after-image

Suppression: Bagolini and neutral density filter bar/Worth 4 dot/4^Δ test

Diplopia: intermittent, in paretic direction, constant, triplopia

Monocular fixation: R/L: central/eccentric. Steady/unsteady.

Localization: Foveal: central/non-central.

Neutral density filter 2.00 log units	VA =	R	L . . . .
Single letter acuity	=	R	L . . . .
Linear acuity	=	R	L . . . .
Near visual acuity (at 33 cm)	=	R	L . . . .

Initial diagnosis

Name of condition(s):

Causation:

Onset:

Treatment

Patient problems	Management	Expected outcome	Actual outcome
(e.g. cosmetic,	1.		
low acuity,	2.		
diplopia).	3.		
	4.		

Discussion with patient/family

See again . . . . . .

Review record

Patient problem	Management	Expected outcome	Actual outcome
1.			
2.			
3.			
4.			

(Complete full record annually).

example of a comprehensive orthoptic record. The P.Q.E. record sheet records the patient's name, age, occupation and refractive correction. Headings are given for history and symptoms, cover test, motility, any other necessary tests, and conclusions and recommendations. The D.Orth. record sheet does not have headings.

5.13   Convergence and accommodation

Measure the near point by 'push up' and 'jump' methods to the nearest 5 cm and check for rapid fatigue by repeating the test two or three times. Measure convergence amplitude by prism bar or variable prism. The normal is 20^Δ or more. It is worth asking the patient to converge voluntarily. Inability to do so may be associated with poor convergence. An additional test of control is to ask the patient to follow the convergence target back again from the near point to 25 cm. This determines whether voluntary control over divergence is adequate. A poor performance may be associated with near vision asthenopia. Record also any symptoms of near difficulty.

It is often convenient to measure accommodation for each eye and binocularly at this point, looking also for accommodative fatigue, lag or paralysis.

5.14   Binocular sensory status

Most squints show anomalous retinal correspondence with a small central suppression area. Those with amblyopia worse than 6/24, or with a large angle over 25^Δ, or an intermittent deviation, or a vertical element post-operatively often show complete suppression. Test with a Bagolini lens (grade two) and neutral density filter bar for distance fixation and the new Mallett near unit or Bagolini lens at 33 cm. The Bagolini lens and the neutral density filter bar are placed before the deviated eye. The patient fixates a spotlight at 6 m or at 3 m. A streak seen through the light indicates ARC. The filter depth is increased until the streak disappears: this is the degree of ARC. For alternating squints two Bagolini lenses are required placed at 45° and 135° before each eye, respectively. The Bagolini lens should also be placed obliquely for vertical and oblique squints.

For suppression, the Bagolini lens remains before the deviated eye. The neutral density filter bar however is placed before the fixing eye. The filter depth is increased until the streak is seen. This is the degree (depth) of the suppression. An alternative technique is to slide a Bagolini red filter bar in front of the fixing eye until the patient reports the red fixation light changing to white or until it is seen in diplopia, one red and one white light. The disadvantage of this technique is that the Bagolini filter bar is graduated in non-parametric (arbitrary) units.

The field of binocular (normal) single vision can be found by recording the extent of version movements binocularly on a Bjerrum screen. The field will be distorted in paresis and post-operatively.

The absence of suppression and the presence of the normal fusional reflex can be shown by a positive *Four prism dioptre test*. With pre-school children, a reliable result may be difficult due to wandering attention and poor fixation. A 4^Δ, 10^Δ or 15^Δ prism is placed base-out before one eye. The child looks at a pen torch. The eye should make a fusional movement towards the apex of the prism. It is easier, however, to watch the other eye make a conjugate movement in the same direction, and then make a recovery movement back to its original fixation position. The test is then repeated on the other eye. Failure of one eye to move indicates suppression of that eye. If neither eye moves, no clear conclusion can be made.

The prism fusional reflex tests

1   *The 4^Δ base-out test*: watch the movement of the other eye, not covered by the prism. Failure to make a conjugate outward movement followed by an inward vergence movement denotes a *foveal suppression area* in that eye. The test may be repeated with 4^Δ base-in.
2   A 10^Δ, 15^Δ or 20^Δ base-out (only) prism may be used instead of a 4^Δ prism. In these cases, look for the inward vergence movement of the eye behind the prism. Failure of one eye to move could indicate *poor relative vergence* or *suppression*. The differential diagnosis between these two possibilities depends upon the presence or absence of diplopia, respectively.
3   *A 10^Δ vertical prism test* may be used in cases of microtropia or heterophoria to determine whether there is more than two Snellen chart lines of amblyopia. This is shown by the absence of an attempted vertical fusional movement in the direction of the prism apex, by the eye covered with the prism.

5.15   Monocular sensory status: eccentric fixation

If the visual acuity of either or both eyes is lower than normal, check monocular fixation (do not confuse with fixation disparity, a binocular phenomenon). Ask the patient to look at the centre of an ophthalmoscope macular aperture, or its fixation graticule. In young children the fixation reflex will achieve this result. If the foveal reflex is in the centre of the stop or graticule the fixation is central. A graticule has the disadvantage of removing the foveal reflex if fixation is on any part of the (black) target. Even if the foveal reflex is not occluded by the black graticule the green filter generally employed will reduce the luminance of the foveal reflex. If a macular aperture is used recheck fixation by asking the patient to look to the top, bottom, right and left of the aperture. Calibrate the angular subtense of the macular aperture by placing it on the optic disc which generally subtends 5° horizontally by 7° vertically. If the foveal reflex is not present record this but estimate its position in the centre of the darker macular area. Record steady or unsteady fixation, or absence of fixation (Table 5.1). In deep amblyopia eccentric fixation may prevent any cover test tropia movement occurring despite an obvious squint. In moderate to deep amblyopia the past pointing technique may be used: the better eye is occluded and the patient asked to point to a target just beyond arm's reach. Failure to point in the correct direction indicates eccentric fixation. Place the image of the ophthalmoscope fixation graticule onto the fovea. Ask the patient if the target appears straight ahead. If not, foveal localization has transferred to the eccentric point. To demonstrate the normal localization of the fovea, close one eye and look at your finger with the other eye. Now look left or right to a new object. The new object is fixated but the original (finger) is still seen as straight ahead (see 4.12).

Table 5.1 Types of monocular fixation.

Central fixation with normal localization
Eccentric fixation with normal localization
Eccentric fixation with eccentric localization
Absence of fixation

5.16   Other tests

Other tests relating to binocular function are listed in Table 5.1 (orthoptic record card). Further details about tests for incomitancy and restrictive paresis, e.g. utilizing tonometry (8.10) will be found in chapter 8.

5.17   Computer orthoptics

Computer programs are available for orthoptic differential diagnosis, for investigation and treatment. One system is 'Computer Orthoptics' (R. C. Instruments Inc, 99 W. Jackson St., PO Box 109, Cicero, Indiana 46034, USA). This was developed by Dr J. Cooper and uses red and blue anaglyphs on a 19-inch colour monitor to measure pursuit and saccadic systems, fusional ranges, heterophoria and fixation disparity, suppression, retinal correspondence, stereopsis and visual memory (Cooper *et al.*, 1986). The Hess Lancaster option measures primary and secondary deviations in paresis, and establishes the paretic muscle.

The targets for the right and left eyes include anaglyph random dot stereograms. The programs can be operated by the patient. The speed of measurement increases and decreases with the patient's response, so forming a type of game. In addition to investigation, there are additional programs for therapy. The investigation programs have been independently validated.

CHAPTER 6
Heterophoria, Vergence and Accommodative Anomalies

6.1   Classification (see also 7.1)

Heterophoria
   Basic esophoria $(D = N)$
   Convergence excess esophoria $(D < N)$
   Divergence insufficiency esophoria $(D > N)$
   Basic exophoria $(D = N)$
   Convergence weakness exophoria $(D < N)$
   Divergence excess exophoria $(D > N)$
   Hyperphoria

Vergence anomalies
   Convergence insufficiency
   Convergence paralysis
   Divergence paralysis (see 9.11)

Accommodation anomalies
   Accommodative insufficiency
   Accommodative spasm
   Accommodative fatigue
   Accommodative lag (inertia)
   Accommodative paralysis

6.2   Causes of heterophoria

Similar factors cause both heterophoria and heterotropia. However the most frequent causes of heterotropia are anomalies of the patient's refraction and accommodative convergence/accommodation ratio. Anatomical factors account for more heterophorias.

Congenital

1   Non-refractive
   (i) muscle insertion anomalies;

    (ii) incomitance, e.g. early paresis resulting in contraction (overaction) of the ipsilateral antagonist which persists after the original paresis has disappeared;

    (iii) A and V patterns.

2 Refractive: e.g. esophoria associated with uncorrected hypermetropia and hypermetropic astigmatism.

3 Partially refractive (and partially non-refractive).

4 Accommodative: due to high AC/A ratio.

Acquired

1 Non-refractive

    (i) trauma or disease of retina (ectopic macula);

    (ii) orbit (space occupying lesion);

    (iii) muscle (disthyroid myopathy, myasthenia);

    (iv) nerve (diabetic neuropathy);

    (v) nucleus (haemorrhage);

    (vi) change in AC/A ratio;

    (vii) change in structure e.g. senile exophoria and reduction in motility;

    (viii) convergence insufficiency.

2 Refractive change

    (i) increase in hypermetropia may cause esophoria;

    (ii) increase in myopia may cause exophoria;

    (iii) increase in anisometropia, producing both sensory loss in the blurred eye and an alteration in the accommodation–convergence relationship.

6.3   Causes of decompensation

Failure of the vergence system of eye movement to maintain fusion adequately in the presence of heterophoria produces 'decompensation'. Decompensation is the loss of control which is present in a compensated heterophoria. Decompensation may only occur briefly under stress or tiredness. Symptoms may be avoided by brief central suppression of one eye. But decompensation may become more frequent and symptoms of tired eyes, 'pulling' on the eyes and stress headache may then appear. Further loss of control may result in symptoms of intermittent diplopia and confusion, with loss of stereopsis, and occasionally, even vertigo and nausea. At this point the motor status could be described as heterophoria/tropia or as an intermittent squint. Finally, 'decompensation' can be used to describe the permanent breakdown of a phoria into a tropia. Decompensation also describes the change which occurs when a longstanding paresis, perhaps acquired in childhood and which has become largely concomitant, once again becomes manifest to the patient, possibly due to the stresses and strains of middle age.

In children, decompensation may produce a gradual loss of stereo-acuity, suppression and an intermittent heterotropia, depending on the age and extent of binocular consolidation. This may happen without any symptoms being reported by the child. In teenagers and adults, decreasing control may produce intermittent diplopia and confusion – the patient may report that 'everything goes into one', meaning two! Brief changes in fixation distance may give some relief, or one eye may be closed during critical visual tasks.

Night driving with the problem of decreased visual information to maintain 'binocular lock', and the effect of fatigue may result in frequent episodes of diplopia. 'Binocular lock' is the extent of visual information which is identical for each eye; in darkness this is greatly reduced, and the conditions are then set for heterophoria to decompensate into an intermittent tropia. The patient may resort to leaving the vehicle interior light on to maintain fusional control. A similar effect may occur when the binocular visual field is reduced, for example, in a recent bilateral hemianopia.

The most common cause of decompensation is transient ill health or psychological stress. Decisions on management are often best left for a few weeks unless there is a history of prolonged symptoms or disability. A new clerical or inspection job may produce symptoms of decompensation. Other common factors include any medication which reduces accommodation, chronic illness e.g. depression, lack of variety in a visual task, discomfort or disability glare and ptosis. In children hyperactivity may be associated with esophoric decompensation and hypoactivity with exophoric decompensation.

6.4   Measurement of heterophoria

The distance heterophoria should be assessed by cover test as to amount and speed of recovery. An accommodative target at 6 m is used unless it is certain that accommodation is not active, when a spotlight is suitable. The correcting prism can be held before either eye to eliminate the phoria recovery movement and thus measure it. The Maddox rod test should also be applied: two tests are better than one. A Maddox rod (multiple groove) incorporating 1^{Δ} base lateral to the handle of a flipper is held before one eye and flipped to establish that horizontal phoria is less than 1^{Δ}. If not, additional prism is placed before either eye and the lens flipped again. The test is repeated for vertical heterophoria with the flipper handle held horizontally. With this technique higher amounts of phoria may be found than with a conventional trial case Maddox rod. For near vision, a cover test then Maddox wing test is used. The Mills Test is a variety of Maddox wing test using smaller sized numerals and thus stimulating accommodation to a more realistic degree. It deserves re-introduction, but a Maddox Wing can be modified to present smaller numerals.

6.5   Measurement of relative vergences (fusional amplitudes)

Relative vergences are also known as fusional reserves, prism vergences (Pickwell, 1989) and fusional amplitudes (von Noorden, 1985). These terms refer to motor fusional ability, and should not be confused with sensory fusion. A prism bar or rotating prism is used to increase prism base-in to measure blur, break and recovery on a distance test chart. A prism bar will increase the prism in jumps, so a rotating (Risley) prism which gives a gradual increase is preferable. Next base-out prism is used to measure positive relative vergence. Vertical amplitudes may also be measured. The measurements are repeated for near vision using small accommodative targets. The result may be plotted on a graph (see 6.6).

6.6   AC/A ratio, and graphical analysis

Graphical analysis is a method of assessing a patient's binocular status. The graph will record the following data (see Fig. 6.1).

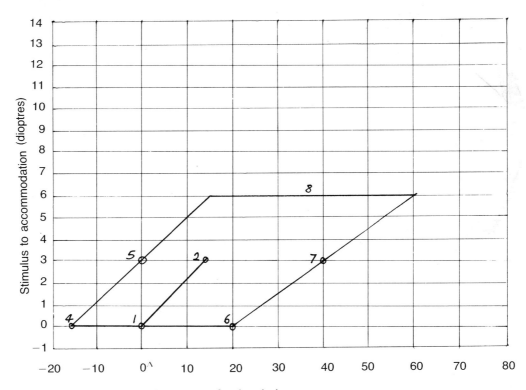

Fig. 6.1 Graphical analysis: see text for description.

1 Distance horizontal phoria or tropia at 6 m is plotted at an orthophoria point 0, 0. If the test distance is 4 m it should be plotted at the position for $+1.5^{\Delta}$.

2 Near horizontal phoria or tropia at 33 cm is plotted from a near orthophoria point at 15,3 so the plot above shows 1^{Δ} exophoria at 33 cm (plotted at 14,3).

3 The AC/A ratio is the slope of the line connecting (1) and (2) here 14^{Δ} in 3 D: a ratio of 5:1.

4 The negative relative vergence measured at 6 m is -16^{Δ}.

5 The negative relative vergence measured at 33 cm is zero.

6 The positive relative vergence at 6 m is shown as 20^{Δ}.

7 The positive relative vergence at 33 cm is shown as 40^{Δ}.

8 Accommodation is shown as a horizontal line at 6 D, connecting the extrapolations (4)−(5) and (6)−(7) so as to enclose the zone of clear single binocular vision.

Following treatment or at a later re-examination, the new data should be plotted in a different colour ink on the same graph so that changes in binocularity can be assessed rapidly. In particular, any significant contraction in the shape or area of the zone should prompt an explanation.

6.7 Fixation disparity curves

Fixation disparity curves can be used to assess whether a patient's symptoms are likely to be caused by a binocular anomaly. The likely response to treatment by exercises, refractive modification and prisms can also be assessed. This technique is popular in American optometry but little used in Europe (see Schor and Ciuffreda, 1983).

The technique of prism adaptation assessment may be even more closely related to symptoms and effective therapy. Prism adaptation assessment is still being developed, (see 3.5).

A fixation disparity curve is plotted on arithmetic graph paper by recording fixation disparity at 6 m and again with 3^{Δ}, 6^{Δ} and 9^{Δ} base-in. The measurements are repeated with 3^{Δ}, 6^{Δ}, 9^{Δ} and 12^{Δ} base-out. The fixation disparity is plotted against the additional prism.

The results are interpreted as falling into one of four typical curves (see Fig. 6.2). Type I shows resistance to fixation disparity over low degrees of positive and negative (relative vergence) demand. There is increasing and equal fixation disparity as the additional base-out and base-in prisms are increased. Type II resists base-out prism induced disparity. Type III resists base-in prism induced disparity. Type IV resists both base-out and base-in prism induced disparity.

Type I which represents 50−60% of the population and type III both

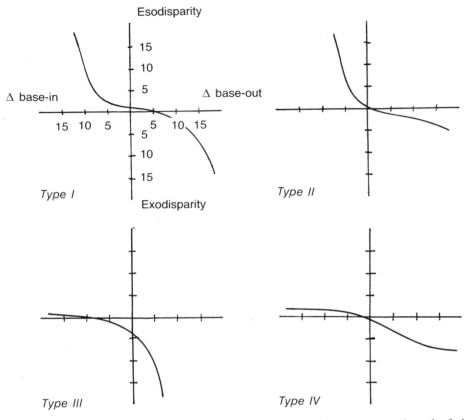

Fig. 6.2 The categories of fixation disparity curves. Diplopia occurs at each end of the curves plotted here. The *type I* curve is flatter in the central area. A flattened curve indicates that the vergence system is able to compensate for the induce fixation disparity (vertical axis) and for the associated phoria (horizontal axis). Further from the origin, the curve steepens, and the induced phoria becomes decompensated. This plot shows an orthophoric patient. In esophoria, the curve would be shifted to the right. Then the portion of the curve cutting the vertical axis would change from flat to steep (in this example), showing an increased risk of decompensation. In the *type II* plot, the esophoria is compensated. Both the associated phoria and the fixation disparity are small. Any increase in esophoria would remain compensated. The *type III* curve shown here illustrates an exophoria which is close to decompensation. The fixation disparity is 4^Δ. The associated phoria is 6^Δ base-in. This is the amount of prism required to reduce fixation disparity to zero and so remove symptoms. With the (rare) *type IV* curve, the patient will have symptoms, even though the curve is flat.

indicate symptoms likely to be associated with a base-line fixation disparity. They would therefore benefit from the therapy mentioned above.

6.8 Management of heterophoria

Management of heterophoria begins by review ('masterly inaction') followed by intervention, with the object of producing compensation including for situations of fatigue or stress which may not occur during a routine examination. Working distance, contrast, lighting and glare, and even blood sugar level (due to missing meals, not diabetes) may need consideration. Next, correction of the refractive error is indicated where it produces a significant improvement in VA or change in vergence demand. Where an improvement in VA produces a disadvantageous change in vergence control, exercises and/or prisms may be needed in addition to correction of the refractive error. Where control cannot be maintained by these efforts, surgery is indicated. The object of surgery is to produce a paresis to weaken a muscle and to strengthen another; a side-effect is to reduce the zone of binocular single vision. Surgery is generally successful in heterophoria because of the pre-existing binocular sensory status. In some cases compensation under all conditions is not possible. In these cases intervention is applied to reduce the symptoms of decompensation or convergence insufficiency. Occlusion is given or else reduction in acuity of one eye by suggestion (hypnosis) so as to allow suppression to occur.

6.9 Guides for prescribing in decompensated heterophoria

Mallett fixation disparity test

Using the distance and near Mallett fixation disparity tests, modify the refractive correction and/or prescribe the minimum prism to align the nonius marks.

Sheard's rule: for exophoria in distance vision

Opposing relative vergence to blur should be twice the degree of exophoria, e.g. a patient with 4^Δ exophoria should be able to tolerate 8^Δ of adduction (strictly positive relative vergence) before a blur or diplopia occurs. If only 2^Δ of adduction produces a blur or diplopia then prescribe $(4 - 2) = 2^\Delta$ base-in split equally before each eye.

Percival's rule: for exophoria in near vision

Percival's rule (the Middle Third Technique): the near fixation point should be within the middle third of the total positive and negative relative vergence range.

6.10   Sensory exercises for suppression in heterotropia

The first two exercises teach diplopia recognition as an aid to breaking down suppression. The third exercise is a possible treatment of obligatory suppression and amblyopia. The fourth exercise treats foveal suppression.

1   *Pathological diplopia* can be produced by bringing a small light source within the angle of a deviation. In this position the suppression scotoma is not usually present and the light should be seen in diplopia provided the patient converges less than the position of the light source. If diplopia is not seen then red and green TNO glasses or motility goggles can be used to demonstrate the different positions of the right and left images. Occlude each eye in turn and upon removing or alternating the occluder the diplopic images should be seen. If they are not seen, a neutral density filter can be held over the non-suppressing eye to produce pathological diplopia. Next the range over which the pathological diplopia can be seen is extended with alternating fixation on a further and a nearer light source. Pathological diplopia is the diplopia produced by a target fixated by one eye and imaged on a non-corresponding point of the deviating eye.

  For distance fixation, diplopia can be evoked by a *Bagolini red filter bar* placed before the deviating eye. While the patient fixates the spotlight at 6 m, the filter bar is moved up in front of the non-suppressing eye going from a lighter to a darker tint to decrease the stimulus to the fixing eye. Eventually two lights are seen, one red and one white.

2   A vertical prism or prism bar can be used to produce vertical diplopia, together with red and green glasses in dense suppression. Having produced diplopia, rotation of the prism (towards base-in for exophoria) will allow fusion — this can be repeated as an exercise.

3   Part-time occlusion of the fixing eye or bi-nasal occlusion of both eyes will stimulate the fovea of the deviating eye and also suspend anomalous retinal correspondence. This can be given where children are too young to do active exercises.

4   *Coloured filter drawing* can be used to treat central suppression. The child has a coloured filter for the fixing eye attached to the glasses and a felt-tip pen of the same colour. The drawing is seen by the poor eye, but the paper by both eyes. The squint angle should be corrected by prisms or by viewing the pen and paper through a cheiroscope. The colour of the felt-tip pen can be changed so as to provide a minimal stimulus for the better eye also, and thus allow binocular vision.

5   A septum may be used to treat suppression in exotropes, using the principle of bar reading. It may be used for distance as well as near fixation distances.

6.11   Sensory exercises for suppression in heterophoria

Physiological diplopia exercises are given, initially using two small light sources (as above) and then two knitting needles or pencils. The targets are held at say 3 and 10 cm from the eyes and fixation alternated (Fig. 6.3 shows a diagrammatic view of the Calder Gillie diploscope, which uses a single nearer light, and at a variable distance, two further lights). A *Lindsay puppet board* (Calder Gillie and Lindsay, 1969) may be used using 2 cm high toys — perhaps three or four on the board and again the child looks from one toy to the other noticing the diplopia (see Fig. 6.4). In intermittent squint the parent should check for bifoveal fixation using the cover test. With improved control, *wire reading* should be possible. The child holds a thin wire midway between his eyes and a book and moves the wire across the text, seeing it in diplopia. When watching television a small coloured light can be placed between the screen and the child — it should be seen double. For exophoria the diplopic targets could be a grease pencil mark on a window and a distance object seen through the window — however, beware of suppression due to glare.

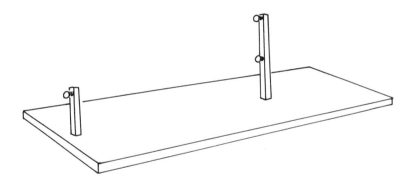

Calder Gillie diploscope

Fig. 6.3 The Calder Gillie diploscope (diagrammatic).

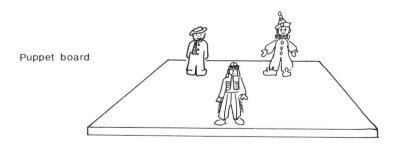

Puppet board

Fig. 6.4 The Lindsay puppet board.

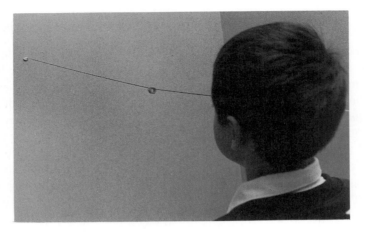

Fig. 6.5 The bead-on-string exercise.

To extend the range of binocular control the *bead-on-string* exercise of Brock, as modified by Pickwell (Pickwell, 1989) is extremely useful (see Fig. 6.5). A string is attached to a wall at 3 m. The string is threaded with a nut, ring or bead and the proximal end held up just in front of the patient's eyes. The patient fixates the bead. The string should be seen in diplopia forming an X shape intersecting at the bead. The bead can be moved along the string away from the patient to extend the zone over which physiological diplopia can be seen and its associated normal binocular single vision. If necessary a bicoloured septum is held vertically at the proximal end of the string to demonstrate diplopia — the red side of the septum being seen by one eye and green with the other eye.

Bar reading is similar to wire reading described above except that the bar is wide enough to occlude part of the text being read and the bar is kept stationary (see Fig. 6.6). The text can only be read if the patient is using binocular vision. The Maclure bar reading book (Fig. 6.7) is particularly suitable, as the text is graded both in size and for reading age.

The *Javal grid* is a variation of this technique. A Holmes stereoscope or a variable prism stereoscope can be used with stereogram cards to treat suppression. The Bradford set of stereoscope cards (see Pickwell, 1989), series F, G and L are suitable for treating central suppression.

6.12   Motor exercises to establish binocular single vision in heterotropia, using diplopia recognition

1   If normal binocular vision ('binocular single vision') is present at one fixation distance, hold a strong stimulus such as a small light source at this position. Move the light away or towards the patient until cover testing shows loss of

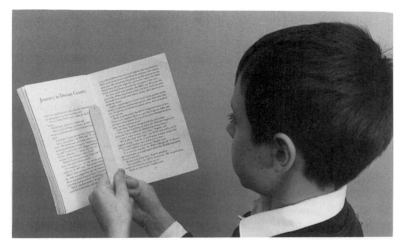

Fig. 6.6 Bar reading.

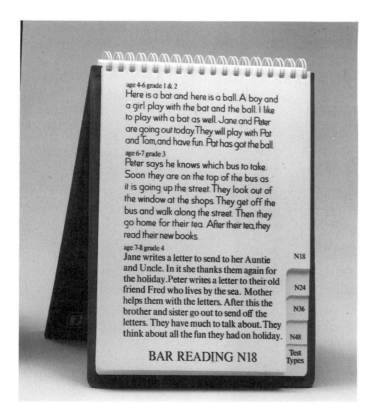

Fig. 6.7 The Maclure bar reading book.

binocular control. If the patient has an A or V pattern utilize the face tilt position (up or down) which provides the best binocular control. The movement of the light is repeated over the binocular zone, in an attempt to extend it. Check with the cover test to confirm bifoveal fixation.

2 *A single mirror haploscope* can be used to extend binocular control − frequent checking with a cover test is again necessary in case the patient lapses into anomalous correspondence or suppression (Earnshaw *et al.*, 1957) (see Fig. 6.8). The targets are a U and an inverted U situated at 1 m. The mirror is rotated to the squint angle and the cover test is applied to encourage simultaneous perception. The mirror may be rotated to provide *macular massage* (see 4.7). The single mirror haploscope avoids the proximal convergence, reduced illumination and small field of view of a synoptophore. It allows a clear view of the patient's eyes for cover testing. A simplified version consisting of a mirror attached to a vertical wooden stick can be given for home use.

3 A prism bar, rotary prism, synoptophore or a variable prism stereoscope may be used in intermittent squint to extend the range of binocular control. In constant squint this is unlikely to work due to a combination of anomalous

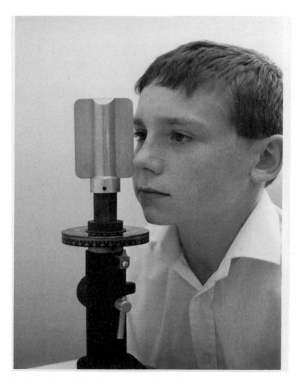

Fig. 6.8 The single mirror haploscope.

correspondence, central suppression and the abnormal visual environment of these instruments.

4   Some control of deviation may be achieved by negative trial lenses to encourage positive fusional vergence, or by having the patient fixate a near object and relax accommodation to produce negative relative vergence − 'looking misty'.

6.13   Motor exercises to extend relative vergences (synonym: fusional amplitudes, prism vergences) in heterophoria

Relative vergence exercises improve fusional, proximal and accommodative convergence in both positive and negative directions, while accommodation is kept constant.

1   *Polaroid vectograms* (Vodnoy) are cross-polarized plastic sheets viewed with polaroid spectacles, as in the Titmus and Randot stereotests. However, the sheets for the right and left eye can be varied in separation and also for different fixation distances. An arbitrary scale at the bottom allows a measure of the extent, and any change in relative vergences from a previous occasion. The targets are a series of stereoscopic pictures which closely mimic vision in 'real space'. An anaglyph version is less satisfactory due to retinal rivalry.

2   The *Bernell aperture rule* is an inexpensive plastic stereoscope which does not utilize lenses. There is a set of stereograms of increasing separation which are viewed through a single aperture to train positive relative vergence and a double aperture for negative relative vergence. This equipment is particularly useful for lending to patients.

3   A *variable prism stereoscope* is a more artificial method of improving vergences. A prism bar is more convenient for home use. The object of the exercise is to allow appreciation of pathological diplopia as a control of eye position. For positive relative vergence, the patient learns to overcome increasing prism base-out.

4   The *Holmes stereoscope* may be used with stereogram cards of varying separation such as the Bradford B, C, D, E and M series (Fig. 6.9). To improve negative relative vergences (for esophoria) the cards are used in increasing separation of pictures, and the adjustable holder can be moved towards the patient's eyes, and the reverse for exophoria.

5   A *synoptophore* or *synoptiscope* type instrument can also be used in a similar way. A synoptophore is particularly useful for improving negative relative vergence, which is slightly more difficult to train using real space methods.

6   *Bar reading* is suitable for improving negative relative vergence because the

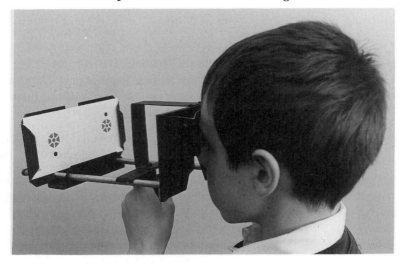

Fig. 6.9 A stereoscope and Bradford stereogram.

accommodation and convergence have to be used together correctly to allow fusion.

6.14   Motor exercises to extend relative vergence in heterophoria

Exercises 1 and 3 improve relative vergence alone, the accommodation being kept constant. Positive relative vergence is exercised to treat decompensated exophoria. Negative relative vergence exercises treat esophoria. The compensation rather than the degree of the phoria is changed.

1 *Bradford stereo cards* series B, C, D and E are used varying the separation with the card holder at a fixed distance. Widen the separation to improve negative relative vergence and gradually narrow the separation for positive relative vergence.

2 Positive relative vergence may be exercised using the *three cats card* or by holding two pencils 3 cm apart at a distance of 40 cm (see Fig. 6.10). The patient over converges so as to fix the left pencil with the right eye and vice versa. Of the four diplopic images the central two are fused. The accommodation is then relaxed so that the pencils become clear − easier for presbyopes. The pencils are then gradually separated, maintaining fusion of the central image (with one monocular image on each side) until the limit of the positive relative vergence is reached. The exercise can be done at different distances within arm's length. The pencils can be substituted by identical strips of text

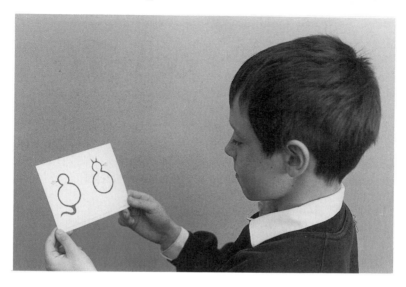

Fig. 6.10 The 'three cats' card exercise.

which should be kept clear — the half page columns from Reader's Digest or similar publications are suitable.

3 *Flip prisms* mounted in pairs on a crossed cylinder type handle can be used to alternate positive and negative relative vergence for a fixed amount of accommodation. The base-out prisms should be two to three times the strength of base-in. Around 4^Δ base-in each eye can be tolerated. If necessary the exercise should be started with a 20 cm fixation distance and this distance increased to 1 m viewing a reading type or equivalent target. The exercise should be done for periods of 2–3 minutes making sure that the text is seen clearly on each flip.

6.15   Motor exercises to extend positive relative vergence and relative accommodation in heterophoria

These exercises use the synergistic help of accommodation for improving positive relative vergence. Later on, the accommodation–convergence relationship can be loosened by encouraging accommodation in the opposite direction to convergence.

Accommodative insufficiency occurs in about 20% of cases of convergence insufficiency. The twin conditions may be transient, possibly due to stress or ill health, but otherwise the prognosis for sustained improvement is not good. To assist with exercises, a bifocal addition with prism base-in may be needed. The reading addition should be calculated in the usual way and the prism assessed with a near fixation disparity test, with the reading addition in place.

1   *Dot card* − a series of 5 mm black spots connected by a black line printed on a rectangular card which is held with one end near the patient's eyes (see Fig. 6.11). Convergence and accommodation are exercised together by looking from the furthest dot in steps towards the nearest dot. Additional help can be given by negative lenses to encourage accommodation. Later the accommodation−convergence relationship can be loosened by positive lenses in front of the patient's eyes thus requiring more convergence than normally associated with the accommodative demand.

2   *Bar reading* as in 6.11 above, but with additional positive or negative lenses to exercise negative or positive relative vergence respectively.

3   *Voluntary convergence* can be taught initially by jump convergence from distance to near vision and back using various fixation distances. Next voluntary convergence without targets can be taught, without which any improvement in convergence may be ill-maintained.

4   Finally, voluntary convergence onto random dot stereograms requires the precise use of convergence and accommodation together with sensory interpretation of a high order.

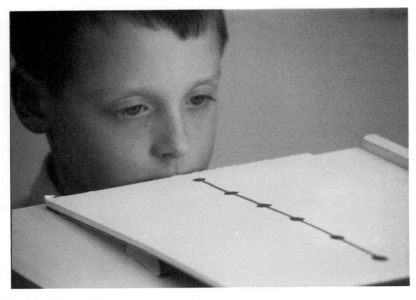

Fig. 6.11 The 'dot card' convergence exercise.

6.16 Motor exercises to improve accommodation in accommodative insufficiency, fatigue and lag (see 6.22)

Ill health, stress and a poor occupational visual environment should be corrected first, if possible.

1 *Flip lenses* +2.00 DS mounted in pairs on a crossed-cylinder type bar are alternated at 10 cycles a minute for periods of 2−3 minutes. The patient views a near test type or equivalent at 40 cm and the text should become clear between each flip. For premature presbyopia a pair of +1.00 DS lenses can be flipped in and out of vision. Premature presbyopia may be due to glaucoma, so check monocular accommodation levels for a significant inter-eye difference. Paralysis of accommodation is associated with mid-brain lesions, convergence paralysis, pupil reflex and visual field changes.

2 *Push-up accommodation exercises* may be prescribed to vary the treatment from flip lenses. They will allow the patient to monitor progress.

6.17 Convergence insufficiency

Convergence insufficiency diagnosis is discussed in 5.13. The patient will be orthophoric at distance and have physiological exophoria for near vision. The symptoms may be merely eye strain where the convergence has gradually deteriorated, but marked diplopia and disorientation for near fixation is evident with a more rapid loss of convergence.

The *management* depends on the presence of associated accommodative insufficiency. If accommodation is normal, exercises should improve convergence. Transient convergence insufficiency may be associated with temporary stress or ill health so the patient should be rechecked when any general health problem has been checked by the general practitioner before starting treatment. Slight degrees of convergence insufficiency may be corrected by increasing the patient's working distance, improving the illumination level, removing glare sources and checking that the condition is not exacerbated by hypoglycaemia, due to missing a meal and rushing to work.

1 The refractive error should be corrected unless minimal.

2 Convergence exercises may be given using a 'pencil to nose' routine provided the patient appreciates diplopia at the limit of convergence.

3 Otherwise, physiological diplopia exercises should be given. The patient looks from a further knitting needle or pencil at arms length to one situated

15 cm closer. The target not fixated should be seen double. The nearer target is gradually brought closer.

4   A variation is to use the Bradford physiological diplopia stereograms (Pickwell, 1989), the orthoptic dot card (see 6.15 above) and prism bar exercises on a near target.

5   The final stage is voluntary convergence. If the patient is unable to converge voluntarily, convergence may deteriorate after treatment. The patient should also be able to follow accurately a convergence target away from the near point.

6   Where accommodation is also deficient, or exercises fail to provide a sustained improvement, prisms may be prescribed. Use a near fixation disparity test at the normal working distance. Any reading addition should be in place before determining the amount of prism required. The prism power is prescribed equally between the two eyes.

7   In extreme convergence insufficiency of 50 cm or so, usually accompanied by reduced accommodation, neither exercises nor prisms may help. Surgery would not be indicated unless there was a marked distance exophoria or tropia. In these cases, occlusion using 'Fablon' or 'Contact' adhesive plastic sheet applied to the back surface of one spectacle lens, coupled with a varifocal lens for the other eye, should be prescribed. This correction would be worn for reading only, unless a distance refractive correction was appropriate.

6.18   Convergence paralysis

Convergence paralysis will be due to bilateral partial third nerve lesion affecting both medial rectus muscles. On testing the near point of convergence, both eyes may lose fixation simultaneously. There may be associated pupil, accommodation and other anomalies. The lesion may not produce exactly symmetrical effects on both eyes. A lesser deficit of convergence, but also with fusion being lost by both eyes together at the near point of convergence, may be associated with a bilateral (nuclear) fourth nerve lesion. The patient will need a neurological opinion in both cases.

For divergence paralysis, see 9.11.

6.19   Accommodative insufficiency

Accommodative insufficiency may be found in association with convergence insufficiency, poor general health due to ocular side effects of systemic medication, or due to disuse, e.g. in spectacle-corrected myopes. Firstly, any general health problem should be treated and then bifocal spectacles or contact lenses prescribed. Any associated orthoptic anomaly should also be treated.

Accommodative insufficiency due to disuse may be corrected with *flip lenses*. For example +0.50 DS and −0.50 DS lenses glazed in pairs. Looking at text at a distance of 40 cm the lenses are flipped at a rate of up to 10 alternations a minute for 2−3 minutes followed by a short break and further repetition.

6.20 Accommodative spasm

The diagnosis is indicated by complaints of blurred vision and painful eyes, myopia, miosis, variable retinoscopic and subjective refraction, or failure of symptoms to resolve with a spectacle correction. The condition is confirmed by cycloplegic examination; the pseudomyopia disappears.

The *management* is to correct the refraction found under cycloplegia with a bifocal addition to inhibit the spasm. Prisms base-in may help to reduce the tendency to go into spasm. Treatment of medical and social problems may help. Later, the bifocal addition can be reduced gradually in some cases. Recently, biofeedback techniques for accommodative exercises have been suggested.

6.21 Accommodative fatigue

This is a mild form of accommodative insufficiency found in debilitated or stressed patients. Bifocals may be necessary. Flip lens exercises are unlikely to help.

6.22 Accommodative lag

A delay in re-focussing from near fixation to distance due to a degree of accommodative spasm is noticed first by patients. Later the delay in changing from distance to near fixation is seen. The normal delay in accommodating is 300 milliseconds so, to produce symptoms, the delay will be twice as long or more. Accommodative lag is a sign of early presbyopia. It can also occur due to ill health, systemic medication, e.g. for hypertension, depression and anti-Parkinsonism therapy or in poor occupational conditions, e.g. night-duty ward sister.

Management: before trying bifocals, the effect of a small base-in prism for each eye should be assessed, as this sometimes reduces near to distance vision accommodative lag. A 'monovision' add of +0.75 DS in one eye may also help to avoid the need for bifocals. The effect, of course, is not monocular vision but binocular vision using a form of the Humphriss technique (Humphriss, 1961). It is only immediately after having a new balanced refractive correction that patients are free from slight degrees of anisometropia.

6.23 Accommodative paralysis

Accommodative paralysis would generally be seen as part of a complete third nerve paresis including mydriasis and ocular motor pareses. Commonly it would be unilateral, and may be associated with aneurysms of the posterior communicating artery or mid-brain abnormalities. Ophthalmic management would include a varifocal spectacle or contact lens correction, but some patients need occlusion to avoid diplopia.

CHAPTER 7

Heterotropia

7.1 Classification of heterotropia

The term 'deviation' includes constant and intermittent heterophoria and hetero-tropia, and combinations of both, for example, at different fixation distances or in different directions of gaze. One example of the latter are incomitant squints, which may be phorias in some directions of gaze, but tropias in others. There are probably more phoria A and V patterns than tropias. It is possible to miss a fully accommodative squint seeing only a corrected hypermetrope with some esophoria. Similarly exotropias controlled with prisms may be examined by the unwary, and the prisms re-prescribed without any suspicion of exotropia being present. Similarly many amblyopes could be more correctly identified as micro-tropias. The moral is to avoid labelling prism corrected patients as necessarily heterophoric. Amblyopes should be assumed to have a tropia or microtropia, unless proved otherwise.

In the following classifications, where tropias are referred to it should be understood that they also include intermittent squints.

Classification of esodeviations

1 Concomitant esotropia
   (i) Fully accommodative
       (a) basic type;
       (b) convergence excess type.
   (ii) Partially accommodative
       (a) basic type;
       (b) convergence excess type.
   (iii) Non-accommodative
       (a) basic type;
       (b) convergence excess;
       (c) divergence insufficiency;
       (d) infantile (onset before 6 months);
       (e) nystagmus blockage (onset before 6 months);

    (f) cyclic (becomes constant later);

    (g) myopic;

    (h) acute (usually psychogenic);

    (i) microtropia esotropia.

2 Secondary esotropia

    (i) Sensory SOT (visual pathway lesion before 3 years).

    (ii) Consecutive esotropia due to surgery, or spontaneous.

    (iii) Esotropia secondary to a primary vertical deviation.

3 Incomitant esotropia

    (i) Paretic esotropia (congenital or acquired).

    (ii) Non-paretic incomitant esotropia (A and V related patterns).

    (iii) Congenital fibrosis.

    (iv) Acquired fibrosis (trauma or infection).

    (v) Retraction esotropia (e.g. Duane's).

4 Esotropia with additional oculomotor disorders

    (i) Congenital oblique overactions which may be unilateral as in elevation in adduction.

Classification of exodeviations

1 Concomitant exotropia

    (i) Basic exotropia: distance equals near deviation.

    (ii) Convergence weakness exotropia (synonym: convergence insufficiency exotropia).

    (iii) Divergence excess exotropia.

    (iv) Simulated divergence excess exotropia.

2 Secondary exotropia

    (i) Consecutive exotropia:

        (a) post-operative;

        (b) spontaneous.

    (ii) Sensory exotropia (onset after 3 years, e.g. due to traumatic cataract).

3 Incomitant exotropia

    (i) paretic exotropia.

    (ii) non-paretic incomitant exotropia:

        (a) A and V patterns;

        (b) fibrosis, congenital or acquired.

Classification of vertical deviations

1 Concomitant vertical deviation: hyperphoria, hypertropia

2 Incomitant vertical deviations

    (i) Paretic vertical deviations.

(ii) Non-paretic incomitancy.
(iii) Dissociated vertical deviations.

Classification of cyclo-deviations

Cyclo-deviations do not generally align themselves when the fixing eye is covered, so a distinction between cyclophoria and cyclotropia is usually made on the basis of any other phoria or tropia which is present.

1 Cyclo-deviations associated with oblique muscle paresis.
2 Cyclo-deviations associated with non-paralytic incomitancy.
3 Intermittent nystagmoid intorsion.
4 Cyclo-deviations due to uncorrected or badly corrected oblique astigmatism.

7.2   Fully accommodative esotropia with normal AC/A ratio

Since accommodation is fully active from 6 months old an accommodative squint can occur from or even before this age. The peak onset age is said to be between 2 and 3 years of age, although there may be a smaller peak around 1 year old. The onset is usually intermittent and more likely to occur when the child is tired or unwell. The refraction of both eyes is generally in the range +2.00 to +6.00 DS hypermetropia and often shows an anisometropia of 2.00 DS or more, or with greater astigmatism in the deviated eye. Few cases occur after 5½ years of age, but occlusion or ptosis in a hypermetropic teenager or young adult can sometimes result in an accommodative esotropia. A common sign is the parent's report of clumsy behaviour, falling over objects or walking into doorposts. Occasionally, the child may close or cover one eye, or more rarely, complain of diplopia. The angle of the esotropia will vary with the room illumination level and therefore pupil size, affecting the amount of accommodation required to provide an acceptable retinal image. The angle is generally greater for near vision and a significant minority have convergence excess − a very dynamic type of deviation in which a large squint may be demonstrated by holding a fixation target at 15−20 cm from the child.

Management protocol

1 The deviation is measured by prism cover test for distance and near vision without refractive correction.

2 Non-cycloplegic refraction is completed and the angle of deviation is measured with the correction in place, for distance and near fixation.

3 A cycloplegic refraction is performed, possibly at the next visit, and the distance deviation is measured.

4   A post-cycloplegic refraction is carried out to see how much of the total cycloplegic result can be accepted without blurred distance vision. The angle is again measured for distance and near vision. If the full cycloplegic refraction is not accepted subjectively try placing 2^Δ to 4^Δ base-in each eye to promote fusional divergence (negative fusional vergence) and see if any further hypermetropic correction is accepted.

5   For children under 5 years of age, the full (cyclopentolate) cycloplegic correction and an additional +0.50 DS may be prescribed. Over 5 years give the full cycloplegic finding or an undercorrection of no more than 0.50 DS. If the child complains of blurred vision, 1% cyclopentolate in single-dose sachets may be prescribed for the parents to instil each morning for up to 3 days.

6   Check compensation, stereopsis and acuity in 1 month. Unequal acuity may be improved by blurring distance vision in the better eye by up to +0.75 DS. If the amblyopia is worse than 6/12, start intermittent occlusion, say three periods of 10 minutes daily while doing detailed close work. A 'Fablon' occluder or a tie-on occluder may be used. 'Pirate patch' stick-on occluders (Bernell Corporation, 750 Lincoln Way East, P.O. Box 4637, South Bend, 46634, Indiana, USA) are popular with children. If stereopsis is below normal and suppression is present, start physiological diplopia exercises for 5 minutes three times a day, or other orthoptic exercises to improve negative fusional amplitudes. Motor and sensory improvement are thus promoted at the same time.

7   Review in 1 month. Recheck funduscopy, motility, pupil reflexes, accommodation, convergence; also visual fields on a screener for children of 4 years and over, or by confrontation for younger children. Use a suitable itemized record card to record the findings.

8   Review at 2-monthly intervals including a repeat cycloplegic refraction at 6 months from the initial visit.

9   At 10–12 years old the refractive correction may be reduced, worn part-time and eventually abandoned if binocularity can be maintained.

7.3   Fully accommodative esotropia, with convergence excess (high AC/A ratio)

Here the full cycloplegic correction straightens the eyes for distance vision, but there is a marked esotropia for near fixation and even more so for a fixation distance of 15 cm. Some degree of convergence excess is found in almost half of all esotropes, but in 20% the effect is readily apparent. The AC/A ratio is 6:1 or higher. About 5% of esodeviations show convergence excess only: esotropia for near fixation but only esophoria for distance. It also occurs purely as a phoria.

Rarely convergence excess may be due to an abnormally low accommodation so that near vision involves an excessive amount of both accommodative and vergence effort: *hypo-accommodation convergence excess*, (see 7.6).

The differential diagnosis should exclude cases of V pattern esodeviation; by contrast convergence excess will occur for near fixation whether looking up or down. Of course, both may co-exist.

Management protocol

1 The deviation is measured by prism cover test for distance and near vision, with and without the full cycloplegic correction. Note that base-out prisms are not normally prescribed in these cases, unless for some additional condition, as they may increase the deviation.

2 Up to +5.00 DS reading addition is given to see if the deviation can be held straight for near vision. The segment should be set to bisect the pupil. Executive bifocals are usually felt to provide the widest near field. In a small child's frame even a 25 mm round segment will cover most of the bottom of the lens. Varifocals have been used but require careful prescribing since they are not primarily intended for children. There is now a Rodenstock bifocal specifically designed for convergence excess treatment in children. Plastic lenses should be given for all children's spectacles.

With an AC/A ratio of 7:1 and a +5.00 DS addition, 35^Δ of deviation can be controlled at near positions. Anti-suppression exercises using physiological diplopia may then be given to extend the range over which normal binocular vision is maintained.

3 Review after 1 month and prescribe treatment for amblyopia, suppression and fusional amplitudes as in 7.2 above.

4 Review at 2-monthly intervals, including any neurological signs and repeat cycloplegic refraction 6 months after initial visit.

5 After the age of 8–10 years, the reading addition may be reduced followed by the wearing time and finally the glasses may be withdrawn, if binocular vision is stable. A proportion of patients require permanent correction in bifocals, and may end up in varifocals or multifocal contact lenses. The provision of a bifocal add of 3 or 4 dioptres to children does not impair accommodation. Typically children have 10 or 12 dioptres of accommodation, and of course they still use their accommodation through the top of the bifocals and even through the segment when using a near working distance less than 25 cm.

6 Miotics can be prescribed to assess the likely response to refractive correction, in particular to bifocals. For this purpose 1% pilocarpine may be used, one drop

in the morning and one drop at midday, for a few days or weeks. The pilocarpine produces an accommodative spasm when near vision is attempted. The accompanying miosis helps to clarify both near vision and distance vision until the spasm has relaxed. Where spectacles or bifocals cannot be worn constantly, for example in a child with extensive sporting commitments, a longer-acting cholinesterase inhibitor such as 0.05−0.125% echothiopate iodide may be used, one drop each morning, the strength depending upon the response. Occasionally a full correction of convergence excess esotropia is only achieved with bifocals and a miotic. Again this can be checked quite easily with 1% pilocarpine. Prolonged use of miotics can produce iris cysts and lens opacities. Parents should be warned that miotics are contra-indicated before (any) surgery, in case they transfer to a different area for an operation. The danger lies in the interaction between drugs such as ecothiopate iodide and Dyflos, and the depolarizing muscle relaxant suxamethonium chloride which is used in conjunction with a general anaesthetic.

The pre-requisites for miotic therapy are: (a) equal visual acuities in each eye, (b) the recognition of pathological diplopia, and (c) a good range of relative vergence (fusion) for distance vision.

Miotic therapy should be used only for 1 month. There is no correlation between the size of the deviation and the effect of treatment. Although the effect of a miotic will be governed by the AC/A ratio, this is of less importance than pre-requisites (a) to (c) above, particularly where the squint is recent (Catford and Wilson, 1981).

7.4   Partially accommodative esotropia, with normal or high AC/A ratio

The largest group of esotropes are partially accommodative: about 35% of all types of strabismus. A minority of these have convergence excess. The residual squint angle with the full cycloplegic refraction in place ranges from minimal to large, with a frequency which steadily falls as the angle increases. Under 10^Δ to 12^Δ the patient's appearance may appear cosmetically acceptable. Over 20^Δ surgery may be necessary.

Primary partially accommodative esotropia

The first type of partially accommodative esotropia has congenital muscle insertion anomalies and hypermetropia. There is often a small vertical element due to inferior oblique muscle overaction which causes elevation in adduction. The onset is usually between 2 and 3 years old.

Secondary partially accommodative esotropia

The second type of partially accommodative esotropia develops from a fully accommodative esotropia with an onset of 6 months or later. Either the failure to correct the refractive error (in the range +2.00 to +6.00 DS) will produce a deviation, or the patient may spontaneously develop a non-accommodative element. Failure to correct the refractive error will, following the squint onset, result in both the sensory adaptations of suppression and anomalous retinal correspondence and the motor adaptation of abnormal motor correspondence. This motor adaptation is necessary to operate a deeply ingrained anomalous retinal correspondence, which requires a small, constant squint angle in all directions of gaze and convergence. Both the motor and sensory adaptations provide a second-class type of binocular vision, but militate against successful treatment. Occasionally a refractively corrected accommodative squint will develop a non-accommodative element and may break down intermittently or constantly. This occurrence should be distinguished from a breakdown due to gradual increase in total hypermetropia. Even an atropine refraction is no guarantee that hypermetropia will not increase, possibly with anisometropia, over a period of years. Therefore a cycloplegic refraction should be repeated occasionally.

Management protocol

1 The deviation is measured for distance and near vision, with and without the full cycloplegic correction.

2 The sensory status is determined using a Bagolini striated lens and a neutral density filter bar, Mallett distance fixation disparity unit at 150 cm, or other suitable tests.

3 If anomalous correspondence is less dense than 0.9 ND using the filter bar and the distance deviation is less than 20^Δ then a trial of *transferred fixation* is worthwhile. The normally fixating eye is blurred by positive spherical over-correction up to +4.00 DS or failing that by a semi-occluding membrane such as Contact or Fablon, attached to the back surface of the spectacle lens. The sensory status is rechecked and if normal retinal correspondence has re-appeared, due to swapping fixation, the patient is given bifoveal stimulation by correcting the deviation with equal base-out prisms. The patient and the parents should be warned of possible disorientation, an indication however of a change in sensory status. Initially it may be necessary to wear the normal correction at school and the therapeutic correction at home. The alternation between the two pairs of glasses should reduce the depth of anomalous correspondence. Amblyopia is treated (see 4.13). Fusional amplitudes should be developed by a combination of physiological diplopia exercises, prism bar, cross-polarized vectogram, stereogram and single mirror haploscope exercises at home.

The blurring should be reduced as the amblyopia improves. The normally fixating eye should be kept at a level of acuity slightly less than the amblyopic eye. Other amblyopia treatment may be given using active exercising of the amblyopic eye for short periods, see Chapter 4.

4 In conjunction with fixation transfer, a trial of bifocal correction should be given. A bifocal should be prescribed, with or without base-out prisms, if it allows bifoveal fixation at near vision, whatever the AC/A ratio. The child should be warned of adaptation problems. These are usually much less than in adults, but a dispensing check within a few days of supply is wise.

5 Anti-suppression exercises such as those involving physiological diplopia or diplopia recognition utilizing vertical prism or coloured filters should be started (see 6.10, 6.12). Fusional amplitudes should be extended using a prism bar, cross-polarized vectograms and stereograms such as the Bradford stereograms, series B, C, D and E. Review the patient at 1 month and then 2-monthly. Do not make hasty changes in refractive correction if the treatment appears to be effective. At 6 months, check visual fields, pupil reflexes, motility and ophthalmoscopy. Cycloplegic refraction should be repeated occasionally.

6 Where the deviation is not controlled by these methods it may be appropriate to go to the next best option. This is to produce a small angle stable deviation with deep anomalous correspondence. The full cycloplegic refraction is given. If any convergence excess is present the near vision deviation should be reduced to equal the distance deviation by a bifocal or varifocal correction. Amblyopia should be treated. It is advisable at the outset to discuss the management with the parents, to give them a printed note showing the object of the treatment, and to record this fact. This treatment regimen can be monitored from the age of 4 up to 10 years. At this point, reduce the distance strength of the correction, and then the wearing time, so that the correction is only used for critical vision. If the anomalous correspondence is deep it should hold the squint at a small angle even without glasses. If not, glasses will continue to be worn, but the reading addition can be gradually reduced. Even with a refractive error as high as 8 or 9 dioptres of hypermetropia, patients may be able to maintain a small angle squint, without a refractive correction. This would only be possible where the deviation had stabilized as a microtropia or fairly small angle squint with deep ARC as a result of fully correcting the ametropia for several years. The ARC may then facilitate maintenance of the same small squint angle, even without the refractive correction. In the late teens or twenties the natural reduction in accommodation will require a partial distance correction.

7   Where the deviation (even with the full cycloplegic correction) is cosmetically unacceptable, around $15^\triangle$ or more, and fixation transfer is unsuccessful, surgery may be required. The patient's general medical practitioner should be given a full report. In patients over the age of 7 years, the possibility of post-operative diplopia can be assessed by fully correcting the residual deviation with prisms. Next, check for residual diplopia on a small light source at 6 m. Instead of using prisms, it is possible to instil a topical anaesthetic and to rotate the globe to the primary position using a cotton wool bud-stick. If diplopia is present when the eyes are straight, the suppression area is too small to include the fovea. Check that the patient's pulse is vigorous and that the rate does not drop significantly during this procedure. The oculo-cardiac reflex produces a reduction in the pulse when the eyes are pressed, or the extra-ocular muscles are pulled.

7.5   Basic non-accommodative esotropia

The term 'basic' means that the angle is virtually equal for distance and near fixation. The onset is after 6 months but mostly before 2 years. Occasionally patients may present with an onset as late as 6 years.

A few children with non-accommodative esotropia occurring between 2 and 6 years have diplopia and do not develop sensory adaptations; they may close or cover one eye. These cases are sometimes referred to as '*normo-sensorial*' esotropia. The mechanism involved is thought to be excessive tonic convergence normally controlled by negative relative vergence, but it is easily disrupted by chronic illness e.g. asthma, emotional stress or injury (including non-accidental injury). In other words when the patient is tired, the central control of vergence is reduced leaving the subcortical centres for tonus in control. Under these conditions binocularity may decompensate.

Patients are sometimes misdiagnosed as non-accommodative when in fact the deviation is secondary to neurological defects including retinoblastoma and intracranial space occupying lesions.

Management protocol

1   If the onset is under 2 years, surgery may be indicated.

2   If the onset is after 2 years and following a careful check for a secondary squint, the refractive error should be corrected, amblyopia treated and then the effect of bifocals and prisms and both together, should be assessed.

The next step is to treat suppression by the appreciation of pathological diplopia (see 6.10). Motor exercises to improve the range of fusion should follow, in addition to the refractive and/or prism correction.

3 Review at 1 month and then every 2 months with a full examination every 6 months to avoid missing neurological lesions.

4 Where non-surgical methods do not have any significant effect on the deviation, surgery may be appropriate. A decision should be made fairly soon after the initial visit.

7.6 Non-accommodative convergence excess esotropia (synonym: near esotropia)

There are four types of convergence excess.

1 Accommodative convergence excess (see 7.3 and 7.4 above).

2 Hypo-accommodative convergence excess esotropia, where over-convergence is due to excessive accommodative effort in a patient with an abnormally low amplitude of accommodation. In these cases any general health problem causing the reduced accommodation must be checked. Possible causes include a generalized viral infection ('influenza'), and the ocular effects of systemic medication. The management is full correction of hypermetropia and a multifocal correction for near vision, assessed by cover test or fixation disparity test.

3 *Non-accommodative convergence excess* (synonym: near esotropia). This type of convergence excess is not due to a high AC/A ratio. The amplitude of accommodation is normal. The distance esotropia is minimal, but the near angle may be 20^Δ to 40^Δ (von Noorden, 1985). Bifocals and miotics are not effective in altering the squint angle. The management is a recession of both medial recti, up to 10 mm, behind their original insertions.

4 Infantile convergence excess (see 7.8).

Type (1) is fairly common and occurs with a fully or partially accommodative squint, or as esophoria greater for distance than near vision, with a high AC/A ratio of as much as 12:1. Type (3) is straight for distance and esotropic for near vision. Type (4) is esotropic for distance and near vision and the management is as for type (3).

7.7 Divergence insufficiency (synonym: distance esotropia)

This is an esodeviation greater at distance than near fixation. It may present as an esotropia or decompensated esophoria at distance fixation and compensated esophoria at near fixation. There may be a small refractive error and good visual acuities. Alternatively there may be a history of treatment of esotropia by surgery which has only partly corrected the deviation, leaving an intermittent or small angle esotropia for distance fixation. This situation arises from the need to avoid a consecutive exotropia.

Management protocol

1 Carry out a Hess plot to confirm concomitancy, particularly the absence of a sixth nerve paresis.

2 Prescribe the full hypermetropic correction.

3 Give a trial of prisms to compensate the deviation at distance. Fresnel prisms may be used or if it is clear that compensation and binocular vision is achieved with up to 5^Δ base-out for each eye, this may be prescribed as conventional prisms and included in the correction. Although prisms may not be indicated for near vision, the patient should be able to adapt to the prisms readily.

4 If prisms do not work, further surgery would be considered.

7.8 Infantile non-accommodative esotropia (synonyms: congenital esotropia, cross-fixation esotropia)

In esotropia with cross-fixation a delay in lateral rectus development results in the right eye fixing for left gaze and the left eye for right gaze; either eye is used in the primary position and occasionally there may be fusion for near vision. Depending on the development of lateral rectus function versus the need to suppress more deeply as visual acuity develops (to avoid diplopia and confusion), the patient may eventually have an esophoria of purely anatomical origin, an intermittent or a constant esotropia. The refractive error is usually low. Other features may include some limitation of abduction, a dissociated vertical deviation, a head turn and latent nystagmus. A form of convergence excess can occur in cross-fixation esotropia (see 7.6).

Management protocol

1 Correct any significant refractive error.

2 Amblyopia is not usually present due to the alternating fixation. If present, it would need treating.

3 If the residual tropia angle with the full refractive correction is over 15^Δ (it is usually quite large), surgery is necessary. This is generally performed between the age of 6 and 24 months in such cases.

7.9   Nystagmus blockage esotropia

About 15% of neonatal esotropias have a special form of esotropia called nystagmus blockage syndrome. On abduction of the right or left eyes a jerky nystagmus appears. On occluding either eye there is a head turn away from the occluded eye. The management is as for infantile esotropia. Surgery produces unpredictable results.

7.10   Cyclic esotropia

A rare condition in which 24 hours of normal binocular vision alternates with 24 hours of unilateral esotropia with deep suppression. Onset is at 4 to 6 years, but after 6 to 12 months the condition becomes a constant non-accommodative esotropia, at which point surgery is usually performed. There may be an associated condition of anxiety, depression, phobia or compulsive behaviour, which may also be cyclic.

7.11   Myopic esotropia

A squint which occurs in children (over -7.0 DS) due to the habit of converging without accommodating, and in adults due to poor acuity associated with high myopia (over -12 DS). Surgery is only indicated if cosmesis is bad; the results may be poor (von Noorden, 1985).

7.12   Acute esotropia

Esotropia may occur suddenly as part of a traumatic paresis. But the term 'acute esotropia' normally refers to a concomitant squint which occurs due to some form of occlusion such as acute ptosis due to injury, infection or allergy, or due to deliberate bandaging of an eye following a corneal injury.

A second type of acute squint (*Franceschetti type*) occurs without occlusion or significant refractive error, but is due to sudden decompensation of esophoria, often with a high AC/A ratio and convergence excess. In this type the relative vergences (fusional amplitudes) are limited and control is lost. Often the precipitating factor is general ill health or social and emotional problems. Treatment may include medication for anxiety or depression, if indeed this is not already being given prior to the esotropia. Correction of the small refractive error and a bifocal reading addition may restore control. These cases are particularly suitable for the incorporation of prisms in the correction, in view of the preceding good binocular control and the usual presence of diplopia, especially for near vision. Children as young as 5 or 6 years old may be affected. The prognosis is good. The refractive correction may only be needed for a few months while the

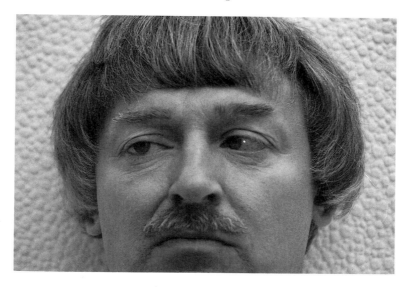

Fig. 7.1 Voluntary squint: left 'esotropia'/right 'lateral rectus paresis'.

underlying factors and binocular control improve. In a few cases surgery may be necessary. Acute esotropia has been reported as part of a severe personality disorder. *Voluntary esotropia* can be learned by children and has been used for ophthalmic training purposes (Stidwill, 1988) (see Fig. 7.1).

7.13   Microtropia

Because there is a complete spectrum of binocular states ranging from bifoveal fixation to strabismus fixus, many definitions of small angle strabismus have been suggested. The term mono-fixation syndrome (Eustis and Parks, 1989) has as its main criterion the presence of a central scotoma in binocular vision, so it includes cases of senile maculopathy and other organic lesions. It is therefore better to use the word 'microtropia' introduced by Lang (see von Noorden, 1985), unless there is also a phoria present. However Lang's definition was almost wide enough to allow the description 'any squint following surgery'.

In common use today, von Noorden's definition of microtropia, or its Latin form 'micro-strabismus' lists:

- **Constant** findings: amblyopia, abnormal correspondence, a relative scotoma on the fovea and/or the fixation spot of the deviated eye, peripheral fusion with some degree of fusional reserve and subnormal stereopsis.

- **Variable** findings: a positive cover test heterotropia movement or no detectable movement, the presence or absence of amisometropia, the degree of eccentric fixation which may equal (microtropia with identity) or may not equal the angle of deviation, foveal or non-foveal fixation response to ophthalmoscopic investigation. The size of the deviation is not included in the definition.

Microtropia 'with identity' is a microtropia where the angle of deviation, the angle of the (ARC) anomaly, and the angle of the monocular eccentric fixation are identical, (see 4.12).

Diagnosis

1   There is a small ($<6^\Delta$) cover test esotropia movement, rarely exotropia or a vertical tropia, with
   (**i**) ARC − sensory adaptation and motor control to maintain a small angle deviation: *microtropia*.
   (**ii**) ARC − sensory adaptation and monocular motor adaptation to the ARC, so that less than the full cover test recovery occurs: *microtropia*.
   (**iii**) ARC and eccentric fixation without identity; the eccentric point lying between the fovea and the retinal area receiving the foveal image. Less than the full cover test recovery movement occur: *microtropia*.

2   There is no cover test movement but the angles of the deviation, of ARC and eccentric fixation coincide: *microtropia with identity*.

3   There is no cover test movement but Amsler chart and Bagolini lenses show suppression, and/or there is reduced stereopsis compared with a previous measurement: presume a *suppression scotoma* in heterophoria. The Amsler grid chart can be used, particularly with reduced contrast produced by tinted or polarized lenses, e.g. the Threshold Amsler Grid (Stereo Optical Co, Chicago, Illinois 6064). A central suppression area would also cause a gap in a Bagolini streak, or when two Bagolini lenses are used, one streak will be reported to be fainter.

4   Exceptionally, where there is no cover test movement, but stereopsis is reduced and/or a central scotoma is present, microtropia can be diagnosed by a finding of anomalous correspondence. This can be achieved in the absence of a cover test tropia movement by getting the patient to report Haidinger's brushes to the side of a target fixed by the non-deviated eye only. Haidinger's brushes can be produced by a commercially available unit with a circularly rotating polaroid filter, the movement of which can be switched from clockwise to anti-clockwise and back. The non-deviated eye fixates a target on a major amblyoscope. Alternatively, the patient fixates a vertical line after-image flashed on the non-deviated eye with a suitably blanked photographic flash unit. A yellow filter should cover the flash window to avoid ultra-violet damage to the eye. A Lee Light Amber 102, or Lee Deep Amber 104 or Lee UV (clear) filter may be used (see 4.13). If the brushes appear displaced from the image a microtropia must be present.

5 The *monofixation syndrome* describes a microtropia which, on prolonging cover test occlusion, shows an esophoria movement.

Management protocol

1 If over 7 years old, correct any significant refractive error otherwise do not treat the microtropia.

2 If between 5 and 7 years old, amblyopia may be treated.

3 If under 5 years old, total full-time occlusion of the fixing eye and full refractive correction will occasionally produce a complete cure of the esotropia with restoration of normal visual and stereo acuity. The patient should be checked at monthly intervals. If no improvement at all occurs within 4 months the attempt to treat must be reconsidered.

7.14   Secondary esotropia

Sensory and consecutive esotropias are discussed here. An esotropia secondary to a vertical deviation can also occur; the vertical deviation is treated first, as in 7.22.

Sensory esotropia

A sensory obstacle to fusion can trigger strabismus. The primary sensory deficit may be due to ptosis, corneal, lenticular or vitreous opacity, maculopathy, retinoblastoma, optic neuropathy including retrobulbar neuritis or a lesion of the optic pathway. Such a lesion occurring in the first few months may cause exotropia or esotropia. From 4 months to 4 years an esotropia is more likely, due to the developing convergence tonus, and thereafter an exotropia as the convergence becomes balanced with divergence and the orbital anatomy develops to produce a divergent position of rest.

Management protocol

The precipitating lesion should be treated and surgery performed to correct an unacceptably large squint angle. An alternative would be to prescribe prisms base-in to give an apparent increase in interpupillary distance.

Consecutive esotropia

Spontaneous consecutive esotropia has been reported (Fitton and Jampolsky, 1964), mainly in a few cases of infantile exotropia which changed to esotropia. Usually consecutive esotropia is the result of an unintended surgical over-correction of exotropia. In a small number of cases the over-correction is a planned procedure to avoid regression to exotropia.

Management protocol

Small deviations up to 15^Δ may be controlled with prisms base-out, otherwise further surgery is necessary where the patient is bothered by the unsatisfactory appearance.

Paretic and non-paretic incomitant esotropias are discussed in Chapter 8.

7.15   Exotropia: basic exotropia

Recent investigation has indicated that some 50% of neonates show intermittent exotropia with decreasing frequency up to the age of 10 months (Sondhi *et al.*, 1988). Those persisting after 6 months may be regarded as potentially abnormal. In addition a number of infant exophores break into intermittent and later constant exotropia during the first year or two. A minority have a squint onset later than 5 years: the gradual onset of myopia in the early teenage years dissociates a further number of exophores. Probably 50% of exotropias remain intermittent. Von Noorden (1985) quotes a series of 51 untreated patients between 5 and 10 years of which 75% showed progression, 9% no change and 16% a spontaneous improvement. Basic exotropia is defined as substantially the same angle for distance and for near fixation.

Management protocol

1   The refractive error should be corrected. Marked anisometropia is best corrected with contact lenses to reduce aniseikonia, unequal convergence and accommodation, and induced prismatic effects, particularly for vertical gaze movements when the eyes look away from the primary position (Winn *et al.*, 1988).

2   Photochromic or graduated tints will help to reduce the dissociating effect of high illumination levels in exodeviations. High illumination levels cause suppression, covering or closing of one eye in intermittent exotropia.

3   Where a deviation can be compensated by a negative addition to the full refraction using up to one-third of the available accommodation or by prisms

base-in or both, a trial prescription should be given (Caltrider and Jampolsky, 1983). The patient should be reviewed at 1 month and 2-monthly thereafter. Exotropes are often asymptomatic and require regular orthoptic assessment to monitor progress or relapse. It is useful to teach the parents to perform a cover test and to record this in a diary between visits. It may be appropriate to give a non-modified refractive correction for part-time use to extend the negative fusional reserve (fusional divergence). Ultimately it may be possible to give the unmodified correction as contact lenses and a prism over-refraction as supplementary glasses for critical visual tasks.

4 Orthoptic exercises to improve positive relative vergence may be worth a trial for 1 or 2 months initially, provided that the family are warned that improvement cannot be guaranteed. The presence of a V or A pattern exotropia is generally a good prognostic sign as binocular vision may already be present in the least divergent direction of gaze. After 2 months with no improvement, the exercises should be discontinued. If the deviation is producing symptoms or is cosmetically unacceptable, surgery may be indicated.

(i) Physiological diplopia, in conjunction with the following exercises.
(ii) Prism bar exercises, increasing the amount of prism base-out and maintaining fusion on a pen torch or fixation spatula at 30 cm, and gradually increasing the fixation distance to 6 m, while the exercise is repeated.
(iii) Polarized vectograms (Stereo Optical, 3539 N. Kenton Avenue, Chicago, IL 60541), varying the separation in both horizontal directions to extend the motor fusion range. The vectograms are cross-polarized and viewed through the same analysing glasses which are used for the Titmus and Randot stereotests.
(iv) Stereograms, used with a stereoscope or a Bernell aperture trainer which uses apertures instead of lenses.
(v) Over-convergence using two pencils, or the three cats card, or the Bradford three cats stereogram.
(vi) Synoptophore vergence exercises or the single mirror haploscope for home use (see 7.16, exercise 6).

5 Adult asymptomatic intermittent exophores are often quite happy if left untreated.

6 Patients with unsightly or symptomatic exotropias do well with corrective surgery because in exotropia sensory adaptations are usually minimal, often suppression or a superficial degree (<0.5 ND units) of anomalous correspondence. Following surgery the original normal correspondence regains control.

7 A significant proportion of exodeviations end up with prisms base-in. They may need two pairs of spectacles because of a variable capacity to adapt to prisms. The stronger prism may be needed when tired or in low illumination.

7.16   Divergence excess (distance exotropia)

In true divergence excess the exotropia is by $7^\triangle$ or more, larger for distance than for near vision. It is often intermittent and may show only exophoria at near vision. A notable characteristic of divergence excess is the variable angle of deviation, depending on general health, anxiety and some degree of control via voluntary convergence. A cover test distance fixation in excess of 6 m will show a further increase in the angle of deviation, as will turning the patient's head to the right or the left. A V pattern for both distance and near fixation may often be elicited by raising and lowering the patient's chin and repeating the cover test. The onset usually occurs during the first year of life. The exotropia is often first noticed when the patient is tired, ill or loses binocular control in bright light (5000 lux). This may be much later than the first year. Sometimes an unnoticed intermittent exotropia becomes constant due to the onset of uncorrected myopia in the early teens. Symptoms are rare but include a heightened awareness of peripheral vision. This is due to the monocular field of vision of the deviated eye showing a higher peripheral acuity than in bifoveal vision when varying amounts of suppression may fluctuate. The sensory status is either suppression or light anomalous correspondence, as normal binocular vision is intermittently present, particularly for near vision.

Management protocol

1   Check the patient's working conditions are satisfactory, with good lighting and minimal glare. Check general health is optimal. A low blood sugar level due to missed meals is likely to produce symptoms and loss of control of an intermittent tropia.

2   Correct the refractive error. Photochromatic or gradually tinted lenses should reduce loss of control in bright lights. The disturbing effects of correcting anisometropia should be minimized by prescribing contact lenses.

3   Consider modifying the refractive correction by up to one-third of the total accommodation present, e.g. −4.00 addition to the refractive correction in a patient with 12 dioptres of accommodation. Assess the fixation disparity compensation after the associated phoria when the patient has worn trial lenses for 10 minutes. Where the modified correction produces esophoria for near vision, or is likely to cause problems with accommodation for near work, consider prescribing a bifocal; better still a varifocal or the Rodenstock Excelit AS bifocal which is specifically designed for strabismus therapy.

4   If amblyopia over 6/12 is present and the patient is under 8 years old, constant full-time occlusion should be given for one month, with appropriate

explanations to the school. Thereafter give occlusion for all non-school activities. Discontinue occlusion if there is no improvement after a total of 3 months. If occlusion is not accepted, e.g. produces asthma attacks, 1% cyclopentolate each morning may be instilled in the non-amblyopic eye for 1 month. Glasses should be worn to correct the refractive error.

5   Both suppression and positive relative vergence may be treated by correcting the squint with Fresnel prisms equal to half the deviation in the right and left lenses. If no improvement in suppression or motor control is evident after 1 month, the normally fixing eye should be fogged by a positive spherical or cylindrical lens to equalize the visual acuities, with the Fresnel prisms applied to the lenses. The presence of ARC greater than 0.6 ND is a contra-indication to this therapy. If the angle is greater than 15^Δ or 20^Δ, eventual control may require operation, and a surgical opinion should be sought before treatment begins.

6   Suppression may be treated by using a single mirror haploscope, which need only consist of a handbag mirror attached to a vertical strip of balsa wood with a flat base to stabilize the device. The patient should wear red and green glasses, e.g. from the TNO stereoscope or red and green Hess goggles. Small light sources are set up at 1 m ahead, and 1 m to the patient's side. The mirror is rotated to produce diplopia. Remove the goggles, place a red filter in front of the fixing eye and rotate the mirror again. Once appreciation of diplopia is present, the filters are removed and positive relative vergence is exercised by rotating the mirror to adduct either eye. The next stage is to use large non-luminous targets, e.g. a U for one eye and an inverted U for the other eye. A cover test can be performed to check bifoveal fixation. This exercise is suitable for home use.

7   Alternatively, a rotary prism or prism bar may be used first to demonstrate diplopia and then to extend fusional amplitudes.

8   If diplopia is not recognized, a vertical prism may be intermittently placed before the deviating eye to demonstrate diplopia. A central suppression area may be treated by tracing, drawing or doing dot-to-dot pictures with a red felt-tip pen and a red filter attached to the spectacle lens of the non-suppressing eye. Only the suppressing eye will see the drawing.

9   Physiological diplopia exercises may be used to treat suppression and improve fusional amplitudes. Two differently coloured pencils or knitting needles are placed in front of the patient and while fixing the further needle the nearer needle is seen in diplopia. If not, cover each eye in turn to demonstrate the different positions of the right and left images of the nearer pencil. If this fails, replace the nearer pencil with a pen torch and repeat alternate covering. The further pencil should be held at arm's length and the nearer at two-thirds arm's length and fixation changed from one to the other. The nearer pencil is gradually

brought in to 10 cm. The synergistic help of a V or A pattern should be used by tilting the patient's head into the position where the best control is obtained, i.e. chin downwards for an 'A' exodeviation.

A useful extension of physiological diplopia therapy is the *bead-on-string* exercise, developed from the original 'Brock string' at Bradford University (see 6.11).

Calder Gillie's diploscope can be used. This has a single light and a vertically separated pair of lights which slide on a metre rule. The Glasgow College version has the lights mounted on two model railway trucks which run on a 3−6 m straight track; this runs along the primary direction of gaze.

Wire reading is a consolidating physiological diplopia exercise. A thin wire is held 10 cm above a book and moved across the text so that its diplopic images straddle the fixation point.

10   *Crossed fixation* exercises may also be used to treat suppression and improve fusional amplitudes, and can be alternated with physiological diplopia exercises to maintain interest. Two identical pencils are held at arm's length about 5 cm apart. The patient converges to produce four images. At first, a finger may need to be held between the pencils and the patient to aid convergence. The middle two images are fused. The pencils are separated gradually, the patient maintaining a fixed accommodative level by maintaining the pencils in clear vision: any text on the pencils should help. As the pencils are separated the positive fusional amplitude is increased. Be careful that the fusion is not obtained by under-converging − this would have the opposite effect. The 'three cats' exercise is another form of this exercise. A card with a picture of two cats is substituted for the pencils, and by over-convergence three cats are seen. The card does not permit any variation in the fusional amplitude however.

11   The *pencil-to-nose* exercise primarily treats convergence insuffiency, not positive relative vergence. However, this exercise can be used as a first step to strengthen the near motor control before tackling the distance motor control − especially when suppression is so difficult to overcome in these cases.

12   *Polarized vectograms* are used, with crossed polarized filters, to improve fusional amplitudes providing there is no anomalous correspondence or significant suppression. The two vectogram transparencies contain monocular markers to check for suppression and an arbitrary scale to record improvement in fusional amplitudes. They have the advantage of providing three-dimensional targets but cannot be used in constant exotropia due to suppression.

13   A *stereoscope* may be used in the later stages of consolidating fusional amplitudes. The Bradford stereoscope cards contain a graduated series of stereo-grams. For motor training, those stereograms with similar designs for right and left eyes are used. The stereogram with the greatest separation is used first in divergence excess and the separation is gradually reduced.

14 In patients with deviations under $15^\triangle$ the effect of prisms should be checked by cover test, fixation disparity test and repeating fixation disparity after 4 minutes wearing of prisms. Failure to adapt to prisms indicates a clinical need for prism or surgical correction. Clearly surgery is preferable for larger deviations or in emmetropia. For smaller deviations and where the patient has a significant refractive error, prisms should be prescribed equally divided between each eye.

7.17 Simulated divergence excess

High tonic convergence type

Complete occlusion of one eye for 30–40 minutes may reveal an increase of the near exodeviation to approximately equal the distance deviation. Before removing the occluding patch, cover the other eye with a hand held orthoptic occluder. Remove the patch and replace it with a prism bar with at least the strength of the distance deviation in place. Perform the prism cover test to measure the angle for near vision using an accommodative target at 33 cm. Equality of distance and near deviations indicates a different surgical approach: true divergence excess may require recession of both lateral rectus muscles. The high tonic convergence type of simulated divergence excess will be treated as a basic exotropia, by lateral rectus recession and medial rectus resection of the deviating eye.

High accommodative convergence type

Measurement of the near angle through binocular +3.00 DS lenses will markedly increase the exodeviation to the level of the distance angle in patients with a high AC/A ratio, i.e. over $5^\triangle$: 1.00 DS. The apparent divergence excess is due to high accommodative convergence. In this case, opinion appears divided as to surgical management. For non-surgical management both true and simulated divergence excess will present a better prognosis than basic exotropia as the patient is closer to good control at near fixation. Also, the variable angle of deviation precludes deep anomalous correspondence. In particular a high AC/A ratio enables considerable manipulation of the deviation with lenses.

7.18 Convergence weakness exotropia

Convergence weakness exotropia is defined as a larger exodeviation at 33 cm than at 6 m. It may or may not be accompanied by 'convergence deficit', which is defined as a poor near point of convergence (>10 cm) and poor amplitudes of convergence (<20$^\Delta$ using a prism bar, rotary prism or a haploscope).

Unfortunately convergence weakness exotropia and convergence deficit are both called 'convergence insufficiency' by some writers.

Convergence weakness exotropia will show normal retinal correspondence at distance with light suppression or diplopia for near vision. The patient may be able to ignore one of the diplopic images, if it is significantly more blurred than the other.

Management protocol

1   This condition responds well to exercises, and failing that to prisms. If there is a poor response to exercises, prisms should be prescribed and the exercises tried again while wearing the prisms.

2   Physiological diplopia exercises (see 7.16) are particularly successful, as are polarized vectograms and the Bradford series of stereogram cards in a Holmes or Asher-Law stereoscope.

3   The amount of prism to prescribe can be found in two steps. First use the minimum prism required to align the near Mallett unit monocular markers. Alternatively use the *middle third* technique of determining the fusional range by measuring abduction to break point (diplopia) with base-in prisms, followed by adduction with base-out prisms, using an accommodative target, in this case at 33 cm. Prescribe the difference in prism dioptres between the dissociated position (angle of squint or amount of heterophoria) and the nearest limit of the middle third of the fusional range. Strictly the measurement should be to the blur point but in practice the break point is adequate and more easy to find. The middle third technique may be used when patients respond to the fixation disparity test by suppressing. A third option is to increase prism base-in until a swift phoria recovery movement is seen upon removing the cover.

4   Next, having assessed the amount of prism as (3) above, it is worth leaving this in the trial frame with the refractive correction for 4 minutes. The 'associated phoria' is then measured using the Mallett near fixation disparity test. If the new 'associated phoria' recorded is similar in amount to the original associated phoria, then the patient has adapted to the prism ('prism-adapted'), and the prism being worn is having no effect (North *et al.*, 1990).

If the new measurement shows a reduction in the associated phoria, then 'prism-adaption' is not taking place — the patient does need this amount of prism. This 'prism-adaptation' technique is said to give a better indication of the amount of prism (or lens modification) required to eliminate symptoms, than the fixation disparity test alone (North *et al.*, 1990).

If there is a poor response to exercises and prisms, and the patient continues with marked symptoms then surgery is appropriate.

5 Where surgery is rejected there remains the ultimate answer to all orthoptic problems: occlusion. Ideally a 'Fablon' or 'Contact' occluding membrane is attached to the back surface of the spectacle lens on the deviating eye. This reduces visual acuity to around 4/60 and allows suppression to occur more readily. The lens is clear enough to render the eye visible to other people — it looks a little greasy. Although in theory only the lower half of the lens needs occluding, in practice patients find this disconcerting and total occlusion is preferable — in which case separate glasses for near and distance vision may be best.

7.19 Consecutive exotropia: post-operative type

In some older patients there may be a history of an accommodative or partially accommodative squint having been corrected by surgery alone. Later correction of the hypermetropia would produce a consecutive divergent exotropia. Cases which occur more recently are due to a cosmetic operation in which patients have suppression rather than anomalous correspondence, marked amblyopia and high refractive error. A small change in residual angle throws the image of the fixation point outside the suppression area, resulting in diplopia. There is an age-related change towards exophoria or exotropia in the general population. In other patients the suppression area is extensive but the slip into exotropia becomes unsightly. Such patients may still show esotropia when their hypermetropic correction is removed, and esotropia may still be present for near gaze, where there is an element of convergence excess. The onset of such a consecutive exotropia may be quite late, e.g. mid-thirties, despite the original operation having been in early childhood. The exotropia will occur at first when the patient is tired and may be some cause of comment by friends, and some alarm. The differential diagnosis could include a recent sixth nerve paresis.

Management protocol

Following exclusion of recent nerve or mechanical lesions, surgery may be indicated unless the deviation is under 15^Δ in which case the patient will merely be reassured and regularly rechecked.

Although surgical under-correction seems general for esotropia, for infantile esotropia with surgery at any age, the best long-term result is achieved by an immediate post-operative angle of 4^Δ to 15^Δ exotropia. During the next 6 months an esotropic tendency produces an excellent result (8^Δ esotropia), which remains stable.

7.20   Consecutive exotropia: spontaneous type

A spontaneous change from esotropia can occur without a history of surgical correction of squint. (In UK hospital practice, the term 'consecutive' is used only for a post-surgical condition; a spontaneous exotropia is classified as a secondary deviation.) In fact, the mechanism may be similar to that discussed above (see 7.19) so it may be difficult to say in a post-operative case whether surgery was a predisposing factor or whether a spontaneous exotropia occurred independently of the surgery.

Predisposing factors in spontaneous exotropia are said to include a late correction of hypermetropia, for example, a small angle partially accommodative squint with symptoms of accommodative stress. Correction of the hypermetropia will reduce the accommodative effort and allow loss of synergistic convergence effort, resulting in exotropia. Other factors would include an unstable anomalous correspondence and a variable degree of amblyopia. Under stress or tiredness, the anomalous correspondence allows the angle to vary and this results in an increase in suppression and amblyopia, to avoid diplopia. This, in turn, weakens the anomalous correspondence further. While active therapy is given, the angle remains small and amblyopia minimal. On discontinuing therapy, both gradually worsen. After a series of repeated treatments and relapses the best policy may be to leave the patient without active treatment. However, the conditions are set for a possible consecutive exotropia.

7.21   Sensory exotropia (synonym: secondary exotropia, symptomatic exotropia)

As in sensory esotropia (see 7.14) deep visual loss in one eye allows a tropia to occur which characteristically may be esotropic or exotropic in the first few months, esotropic thereafter up to 4 years and exotropic where the visual loss occurs after 4 years.

Management protocol

The primary cause of the visual loss is treated where possible and squint surgery is given for cosmetic improvement. A common type of sensory exotropia is due to unilateral traumatic cataract in a young child. The cataract is removed, a contact lens is fitted, and orthoptic treatment is given to reduce the rapid development of amblyopia and suppression. However, unless a bifocal contact lens is supplied, or bifocal or varifocal spectacles, the chances of a binocular result are not high since most of a child's critical visual tasks are at quite close working distances.

Paretic and non-paretic incomitant exotropias are discussed in Chapter 8.

7.22 Vertical deviations: concomitant hyper/hypotropia

Vertical deviations are rarely fully concomitant. Of those which are concomitant, the cause may be orbital dysymmetry, abnormal orbital ligaments or abnormal innervation, e.g. neural hypotrophy. Other cases may have been originally incomitant but became concomitant over a period of time. The sensory status is usually suppression or intermittent diplopia. Of the smaller deviations, about half show vertical anomalous correspondence. Asymptomatic patients show large vertical fusional amplitudes. Symptomatic cases may have small vertical fusional reserves and intermittent diplopia which can be less readily ignored than horizontal diplopia.

Management protocol

1 Check concomitancy by motility using a small non-focussed light source or by Hess plot.

2 Check for cyclodeviations by red and white vertical Maddox rods. Bagolini lenses can be used vertically but if fused at an inclination to each other will produce a single streak of light which is tilted antero-posteriorly.

3 If the patient reports symptoms or poor cosmetic appearance, prescribe prism using a fixation disparity test, or (failing that) by the minimum prism to achieve a rapid cover test recovery on removal of the occluder. The vertical deviation should be measured after wearing the prism for 4 minutes. Then if the deviation measurement is the same (ignoring the prisms in position) as it was originally, the patient has adapted to the prism and would appear not to need that amount of prism. If there are symptoms, repeat with a larger prism correction. The prism should be prescribed equally divided between the two eyes.

4 Patients will generally accept any amount of prism including Fresnel prisms, which remove diplopia.

5 If prisms are unsuccessful, surgery by lifting or lowering the insertions of horizontal muscles can be performed to correct up to 12^Δ (von Noorden, 1985).

7.23 Dissociated vertical deviation (synonyms: dissociated vertical divergence, alternating sursumduction, 'DVD')

The synonym of 'alternating sursumduction' is inappropriate since excyclotorsion is also present. The term 'divergence' is best left to horizontal anomalies. The diagnosis made by occluding each eye in turn. The occluded eye moves upwards under cover in each case (see Fig. 7.2). While one eye is covered, a neutral

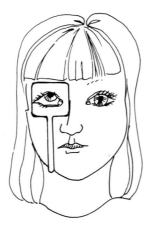 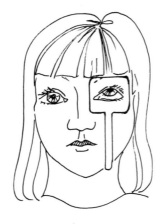

Fig. 7.2 Dissociated vertical deviation.

density filter bar is placed before the fixing eye. As the filter depth is increased, the other (covered) eye will move down. A third test can be performed by moving a Teller Acuity card rapidly (20 degree/second) from left to right and back. In DVD, optokinetic nystagmus only occurs in one direction in patients who also have horizontal heterotropia, i.e. nasalward (Mein, 1983). Latent nystagmus occurs in about half of all DVD patients and rarely otherwise (von Noorden, 1985). DVD may occur in the absence of any other binocular anomaly but commonly occurs with concomitant and incomitant squints. DVD may be superimposed on a vertical tropia or phoria. Occasionally DVD appears when the patient is tired or ill. These patients often have large vertical amplitudes.

Management protocol

1   Any concurrent binocular anomaly should be treated.

2   DVD may often spontaneously improve.

3   Surgery is not normally given.

7.24   Cyclodeviations

A cyclodeviated eye remains intorted or extorted under both monocular and binocular conditions. Conventionally it is called cyclophoria if any associated oculomotor anomaly is a phoria, and cyclotropia if there is also a horizontal or vertical tropia.

Cyclodeviations are found in A and V patterns, dissociated vertical deviations and with paresis, generally of the oblique muscles. They are said to occur in medium to high uncorrected oblique astigmatism or where the correcting cylinder is at the wrong axis. Torsional diplopia and oscillopsia can occur in superior oblique myokymia (tremor).

Management protocol

1   Correct any medium to high astigmatism.

2   Check the axis of current spectacle correction and especially toric contact lenses.

3   Check for paresis.

4   Correct any associated vertical tropia or phoria with prisms. This may reduce the cyclodeviation and allow cyclofusion (mainly a sensory faculty) to occur.

5   Cyclofusional amplitudes may be developed using a synoptophore, or by rotating a pair of white or red Maddox rods in the opposite direction to the deviation. The patient should be warned of possible vertigo or nausea.

6   If the patient still has symptoms, surgery may be appropriate, usually of the oblique muscles.

7   Occlusion can be given for intractable diplopia.

8   It is possible, experimentally, to correct cyclotropia with Ames' cyclotropia tilted mirror spectacles.

CHAPTER 8
Incomitancy

8.1   Non-paretic versus paretic incomitancy

Incomitancy consists of a conflict between version control, and fusional vergence control. It results in a tendency for the extra-ocular muscles to over- or under-act in particular directions of gaze. It presents as a heterophoria or heterotropia which increases as the eyes make a version movement into the incomitant direction of gaze. In non-paretic incomitancy the deviation remains the same whichever eye fixates (Table 8.1). In paresis the deviation is greater when the paretic eye is fixing because there is a marked overaction of the good eye. Later a 'spread of concomitance' occurs (Table 8.2). In recent paresis, the fixation object appears further from the primary direction than it actually is, when the affected eye is looking monocularly in the direction of action of the paretic muscle. So if the patient is asked to locate the fixation object, he 'past-points'.

In restrictive (mechanical) paresis, movement may be limited in opposing directions (see 8.10). For example, a fibrosed lateral rectus muscle will neither contract for dextroversion, not relax for laevoversion. The result may be an 'up-

Table 8.1 Differential diagnosis: paretic/non-paretic incomitancy.

	Non-paretic	Paretic
Diplopia	Uncommon	Common
Onset	Congenital	Later
Primary less than secondary deviation	No	Yes
Head Position	Up or down in A/V patterns, otherwise straight.	Tilt and or turn
Head injury	No	Common
Neurological or systemic disease	No	Possible

I18

Table 8.2 Differential diagnosis: old versus new paresis.

Presence of diplopia
  Old: No, except decompensation of old paresis previously controlled by heterophoria
  New: Yes — in affected direction of gaze

Effect of diplopia
  Old: Minor problem to patient
  New: Often a major problem

Overaction of contralateral synergist
  Old: Overaction similar in extent to underaction of affected muscle, but greater
        overaction if an abnormal head posture is present
  New: Large overaction, greater than underaction of paretic muscle

Symptoms
  Old: None, unless recent decompensation has occurred
  New: May be symptoms of intracranial lesion or systemic disease

Abnormal head position
  Old: May persist on occluding paretic due to secondary orthopaedic torticollis
  New: Disappears on occluding paretic eye

shoot' or 'down-shoot' during an intended purely horizontal eye movement, or a retraction of the eye into the orbit. 'Up-' and 'down-shoots' occur when a muscle slips obliquely over the globe, and can occur as a primary overaction (see 8.3) or secondarily (see 8.10).

An example to illustrate the development of a paresis follows.

Stage 1: At onset: Recent *paresis* of RSR (perhaps due to injury or diabetic neuropathy) — underaction of RSR up and to the right with diplopia — right hypotropia in that direction.

Stage 2: 1 week later: *overaction* of LIO (the contralateral synergist). This follows from Hering's Law. When looking up and to right, the deviation increases, diplopia widens and is more obvious to the patient. Right hypotropia increases and is evident over the whole upper right quadrant of the binocular field of vision. The LIO overaction will be more noticeable than the RSR underaction.

Stage 3: 1 month later: *contracture* of the ipsilateral antagonist RIR — this causes the diplopia to widen further, and right hypotropia affects the whole of right gaze. (This follows from Sherrington's Law.) This contracture produces a greater deviation angle than the original purely paretic deviation. At this stage, diplopia may be widest down and to the right. If this contracture can be avoided, for instance by alternate occlusion coupled with motility exercises, or by Botulin toxin injection (see 8.9) or by prescribing a prism to allow the patient to regain binocular control coupled with physiological diplopia exercises in the affected direction of gaze, the prognosis will be improved. Otherwise the contracture may develop, with the accompanying reduction of elasticity of the contracted muscle. This causes a later increase of the primary deviation to equal the secondary deviation. However, at this point, the affected eye can no longer reach the mid-line. Originally the movement of the paretic eye would be restricted only in the field of action of the paretic muscle.

Stage 4: 2 months later: *secondary inhibitional paresis* of the contralateral antagonist, the LSO. (This follows from Hering's Law.) The LSO may be mistaken as the primary paresis: this can be checked by the Parkes three-step test (see Table 8.3), or by cover test looking right and then left.

Stages 3 and 4 may not always occur if the patient habitually fixates with the paretic eye — due to strong ocular dominance or incipient cataract in an older patient: beware the ancient examination subject who may well be in this situation!

The time scales given for stages 1 to 4 can be widely different, depending upon the original cause, and subsequent management. The 'spread of concomitance' may entirely mask the signs of paresis, thus concealing the paretic origin of some apparently concomitant non-accommodative squints.

8.2   Non-paretic incomitancy

Small degrees of incomitancy are commonly found during the routine examination of ophthalmic patients. This is particularly so if diplopia is sought at the

Table 8.3 Parks three-step test for vertical paresis diagnosis.
(developed from the Bielschowsky head tilt test, Hofmann and Bielschowsky, 1900)

Step 1: Has the patient a right or left hypotropia? (Classify a hypotropia as a hypertropia of the opposite eye)
Although a Hess screen plot normally provides all the information necessary to diagnose muscle under and overactions, the Parks three-step test is a further aid in distinguishing between a vertically acting muscle which is primarily underacting, from one which is secondarily underacting. It is more reliable in a fairly recent paresis, rather than a very long-standing paresis.

RIGHT HYPERTROPIA	LEFT HYPERTROPIA
RSO,RIR,LIO,LSR	RIO,RSR,LSO,LIR

Step 2: Is the hypertropia greater in right or left gaze?

RIGHT GAZE	LEFT GAZE
RSR,RIR,LIO,LSO	LSR,LIR,RIO,RSO

Step 3: Is the hypertropia greater with head tilt to the right or left?

RIGHT TILT	LEFT TILT
RSO,RSR,LIO,LIR	RIO,RIR,LSO,LSR

Which muscle is common to steps 1, 2 and 3?: the paretic muscle

---

extremes of eye movement. Overaction of one inferior oblique muscle, elevation in adduction, is the most frequently seen incomitancy. The causes include anatomical variations in orbital shape as in Apert's and Crouzon's syndromes, the extent of check ligaments, the insertion of muscle tendons onto the globe and the adherence of extra-ocular muscles to themselves or surrounding tissue.

8.3 Overaction of the inferior oblique muscle

On horizontal motility testing, one eye may move first towards the nose, as expected, but may then make a jerky 'upshoot'. This is known as 'elevation in adduction'. It can be unilateral or bilateral, and is a primary overaction, not to be confused with a secondary inferior oblique overaction associated with a contralateral superior rectus paresis (in which case a vertical tropia will be present in the primary position). The cause may be a structural anomaly in the fascia surrounding the insertions of the inferior oblique and medial rectus, or due to reduced tonus in the ipsilateral superior oblique, where esotropia is present. Inferior oblique overaction can occur independently or associated with infantile esotropia, exotropia and V pattern incomitancy. Other 'up-' and 'down-shoots' are seen in restrictive paresis (see 8.10).

8.4 A and V pattern incomitancy

About one in four strabismus patients shows a marked change in horizontal deviation as distance fixation changes from looking 30° up to looking 30° down. The definition is a $10^\triangle$ change for A pattern and $15^\triangle$ for V pattern. The incidence in the non-strabismic population is also high (in the author's experience, about 10% of non-strabismic ophthalmic patients show a V pattern). A $5^\triangle$ V pattern is regarded as physiological (von Noorden, 1985). These patterns are, in order of frequency, V esotropia, A esotropia, V exotropia and A exotropia. In some cases the change may convert an esotropia to an exotropia as the vertical eye movements are made (an X pattern). The cover test should be performed with the head tilted back, and then forward. In addition to cover testing at distance and near, a Hess plot should be made.

The *aetiology of A and V patterns* is not agreed and may vary in individual patients. Over and underaction of the oblique muscles appears to be the most likely cause (see Table 8.4). In the primary position, both superior and inferior obliques provide an element of abduction. A and V patterns occur with:

1 Abnormal insertions of the horizontal recti (i.e. too high or too low).
2 Abnormal insertions of the oblique muscles (i.e. too posterior or too anterior).
3 Secondary to the torsional effects of the oblique muscles (i.e. causing the ipsilateral antagonist to overact).
4 Due to secondary horizontal actions of the vertical recti (i.e. causing the synergist oblique muscle to overact).

Table 8.4 Oblique muscle actions.

Muscle	Primary action	Secondary	Tertiary
Superior oblique	Incycloduction	Depression	Abduction
Inferior oblique	Excycloduction	Elevation	Abduction

Note that while diplopia may be found when looking up, or down, the images will be *horizontally* separated.

If the superior oblique underacts its abduction will fail and the eye will move nasally, especially in depression when the maximum action is normally achieved. Superior oblique underaction will also produce contracture of the ipsilateral antagonist (see 8.1): the inferior oblique. This secondary overaction of the inferior oblique will include additional abduction, particularly in elevation – the maximum field of action of this muscle. The eye will therefore move temporally in upgaze.

These two effects comprise a V pattern. An A pattern would be produced by weakness of the inferior oblique muscles and secondary overaction of the superior obliques.

A primary overaction could explain the Y and inverted Y variations. A and V patterns in some cases may be due to primary underaction of the superior or inferior recti causing a secondary over or underaction of the oblique muscles. The importance of A and V patterns is that binocular vision may be retained in some directions of gaze, and also deep sensory adaptations are less likely with such a variable squint angle. The prognosis for both conservative and surgical treatment is therefore good. Non-surgical management includes the use of oblique prisms, vertical prisms and bifocals where the AC/A ratio is high enough to reduce a deviation, particularly where a refractive correction will be a permanent requirement anyway. Fusional vergences (amplitudes) may be improved (see 6.12 and 6.13). Where these measures do not produce a reasonable control for normal working distances and head positions, surgery may be indicated.

8.5   Neurogenic paresis

Congenital neurogenic paresis can be due to isolated familial hypotrophy of a nerve or its nucleus. Rarely it can be associated with major brain abnormalities. A congenital paresis may be held in check by a head tilt or turn and by well developed fusional amplitudes until some transient illness or increasing stress and tiredness produces a loss of control and diplopia. This decompensation may occur when the patient reaches the thirties or forties. Childhood photographs may show ocular torticollis. Acquired neurogenic paresis most frequently affects the sixth cranial nerves (because of their susceptibility to raised intracranial pressure as they pass over the petrous portion of the temporal bones), and the fourth and third nerves less often. The paresis may encourage the development of a horizontal or vertical squint which may persist after the spread of concomitance has obscured the paresis. In particular, transient sixth nerve paresis due to a head injury may result in esotropia which may be non-accommodative or partially accommodative. Acquired neurogenic paresis in some cases may be associated with pain around the eye and headache in diabetic neuropathy, Gradenigo's syndrome, herpes zoster, sinusitis and temporal arteritis.

8.6   Sixth nerve paresis

In children a sixth nerve neurogenic paresis can be caused by birth trauma and transient episodes of meningitis and pyrexia (see Fig. 8.1). Birth trauma involves the sixth nerve by increased intracranial pressure which presses the nerve against the petrous temporal bone. The diminished nerve function is probably caused by a local reduction in blood supply where the pressure increase is gradual, and may be reversible. A sudden increase in pressure, as in trauma, will cause immediate direct damage to the nerve. Some recovery of function may still occur, and continue over a period of 9 months or so. A low-grade encephalitis such as that produced by an upper respiratory tract infection with the additional symptom of headache can produce shortlived diplopia (and dysarthria). Transient sixth nerve diplopia can also accompany meningism (meningeal irritation causing a stiff neck or pain on attempted head movement) in acute fever, meningitis, otitis

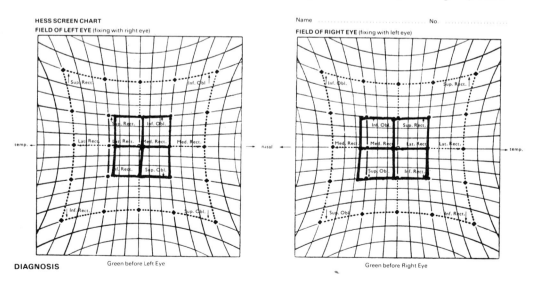

Fig. 8.1 Hess plot. Old neurogenic LLR paresis − sixth nerve lesion.

media, and pneumonia. A bilateral sixth nerve lesion will result in cross-fixation. The slower the recovery the greater the damage — in the form of non-accommodative esophoria, intermittent esotropia, unilateral or alternating esotropia, in that order.

In the patient's working life the major causes of sixth nerve paresis are trauma, demyelinating disease and intracranial space occupying lesions, while in old age cerebral vascular accidents are more common. A lesion of the sixth nerve nucleus must also produce gaze-paresis to the same side. Further down the nerve pathway Gradenigo's syndrome can occur. This acquired syndrome occurs with meningitis, and osteitis at the tip of the petrous bone, usually following a mastoid or middle ear infection on the same side. It produces a sixth nerve paresis with pain and deafness on the affected side. Within the cavernous sinus, aneurysms, haemorrhage and pituitary tumours may involve the third, fourth, fifth and sixth nerves. Continuing down the nerve, head trauma involving a hairline fracture around the superior orbital fissure and optic foramen can also involve the second nerve with some degree of unilateral hemianopia. Finally orbital cellulitis may add the further complications of proptosis and pain on eye movement. Transient cellulitis is not uncommon in general practice with a reduction in acuity and orbital tenderness on palpation lasting 1 or 2 days, perhaps associated with a minor viral infection, e.g. influenza or an upper respiratory tract infection. The differential diagnosis, however, includes orbital tumours.

8.7   Fourth nerve paresis

Congenital fourth nerve neurogenic paresis may be due to hypoplasia or haemorrhage (see Fig. 8.2). Either can affect both fourth nerve nuclei producing a V pattern. The Hess plot of course is made with the two eyes making version, not vergence movements. Thus a fourth nerve lesion can simultaneously produce a V pattern but also some degree of convergence insufficiency — the superior oblique muscle is known as the 'reading muscle'. Acquired fourth nerve paresis is commonly traumatic but can also be due to those factors affecting the sixth nerve (see 8.6).

The Hess plot is usually conclusive but in patients who do not co-operate adequately the Parkes three step test (based on the Bielschowsky head tilt test) may be needed to distinguish a superior oblique from a superior rectus paresis of the opposite eye. This is because the superior rectus is the contralateral antagonist. It may show the final motor sequel: secondary inhibitional paresis. The original superior oblique underaction may have become less evident. A simplified head tilt test, where there is a choice of these two muscles to check whether the hypertropia increases upon tilting the head to the paretic side, is useful. If it does increase, a superior oblique paresis is confirmed. A superior oblique paresis

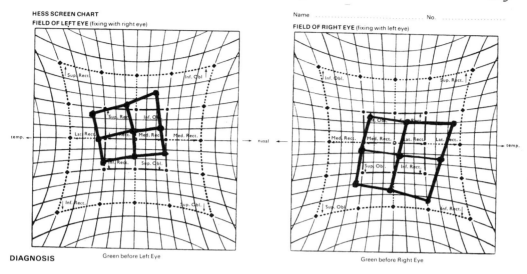

Fig. 8.2 Hess plot. Recent neurogenic LSO paresis – fourth nerve lesion.

is the most common cause of a head tilt. Intermittent oscillopsia following a fourth nerve paresis is due to benign superior oblique myokymia.

8.8 Third nerve paresis

Congenital third nerve neurogenic paresis may be caused by birth injury. Trauma is a major cause of acquired third nerve paresis in children. Head injury, diabetic vascular disease and aneurysms of the circle of Willis (especially posteriorly) are the main causes of third nerve paresis in adults (see Figs 8.3 and 8.4). In later life hypertension can also cause this lesion.

During recovery from extensive third nerve damage aberrant nerve regeneration of nerve fibres can result in unilateral lid lag and occasionally miosis when the eye moves downwards. The existence of an intermittent third nerve paresis has been reported: *cyclic paresis*.

Third nerve neurogenic paresis types

1 Complete paresis – both extra- and intra-ocular muscles
2 Partial paresis
  (i) extra-ocular muscles only.
  (ii) superior division of third nerve – superior rectus and levator palpebris.
  (iii) inferior division – IR, MR, IO, sphincter, ciliary muscle.
  (iv) combined superior and inferior division: SR and IO (double elevator paresis).

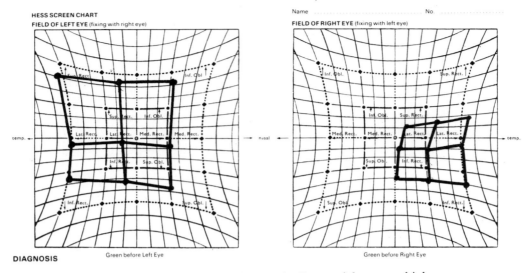

Fig. 8.3 Hess plot: third nerve neurogenic paresis. Recent right eye multiple pareses.

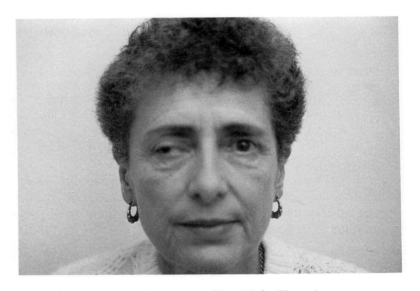

Fig. 8.4 Recent right third nerve lesion — see Fig. 8.3 for Hess plot.

3   Single muscle paresis (usually congenital)
    (i) superior rectus with V pattern exotropia.
    (ii) medial rectus.
    (iii) inferior rectus (least common).

An acquired superior rectus paresis will generally be accompanied by ptosis since the superior and levator share the superior division of the third nerve, and also are anatomically in close proximity.

8.9 Multiple neurogenic paresis (subnuclear and nuclear)

For pareses associated with internuclear and supranuclear lesions, see chapter 9. The effects of double elevator and double depressor pareses are described in Table 8.5. Some syndromes which involve multiple neurogenic pareses are shown in Table 8.6.

Table 8.5 Double elevator and depressor pareses.

Name	Muscles	Effect
Double elevator	Superior rectus and Inferior oblique	Non-paretic eye fixing: paretic eye is hypotropic, with ptosis Paretic eye fixing: non-paretic eye: hypertropic, ptosis goes
Double depressor	Inferior rectus and Superior oblique	Non-paretic eye fixing: paretic eye is hypertropic in primary position Paretic eye fixing: non-paretic eye is hypotropic in primary position

Table 8.6 Syndromes involving multiple neurogenic pareses.

Name of syndrome	Lesion	Effect
Benedikt	III and red nucleus	Exotropia on same side as lesion, contralateral intention tremor of arm and leg
Foville	VI and VII nuclei	Lateral rectus paresis
Millard-Gubler	VI, can affect VII	Ipsilateral esotropia and facial paralysis. Cross hemiplegia
Moebius	VI and VII	Esotropia, Bell's phenomenon, facial paralysis, tongue and hand anomalies
Weber	III and pyramidal tract	Medial rectus paresis and exotropia on same side as lesion. Cross hemiplegia
Wernicke	VI, and may affect III and IV (due to alcoholism and other malnutritional states)	Lateral rectus paresis, complete external (and occasional internal) ophthalmoplegia, nystagmus, ataxia and ptosis

Management protocol

1 The underlying cause of the paresis should be investigated and treated where appropriate.

2 The contracture of the ipsilateral antagonist which occurs within a period of weeks may be avoided by giving convergence and divergence exercises in the field of the muscles action adjacent to the diplopic area, but where control is still retained. The exercises are gradually brought further towards the field of action of the paretic muscle.

3 After any spontaneous improvement has occurred during the first 6 months, injections of botulin toxin are made into the ipsilateral antagonist. There is evidence that this procedure is beneficial for medial rectus injections following lateral rectus paresis (Scott, 1981).

4 Prisms base-out in front of the non-paretic eye have been advocated for lateral rectus paresis, to avoid medial rectus contracture (Guibor, 1950). However, no evidence of benefit has been shown so far.

5 For lesser degrees of paresis no treatment may be necessary since, when an eye movement over $10°$ (17^Δ) is made, a head movement is also made and this may be sufficient to avoid diplopia. Diplopia in extreme eye positions, particularly superiorly, does not usually present problems to the patient.

6 A recent appearance of paretic diplopia with no other signs or symptoms may be due to decompensation of the relative vergences (fusional amplitudes), due to stress or tiredness or a transient illness. If a low degree of prism removes the diplopia and then a larger than normal relative vergence is found, particularly if a vertically acting muscle is involved, this raises a presumption of a decompensation of a long-standing paresis.

7 Prisms may be prescribed to cover the whole or part of a spectacle lens, or serially, using Fresnel prisms. Serial Fresnel prisms are applied in 4 mm wide strips, increasing by 2^Δ steps across all or part of a spectacle lens. They work best for horizontal pareses.

For a bilateral lateral rectus underaction 2^Δ to 4^Δ base-out each eye (over the whole of each lens) may be prescribed to remove diplopia on either side. Prism adaptation allows retention of binocular single vision in the primary and converged positions.

8 In a recent paresis there is a spread of concomitance which takes $6-8$ months to stabilize. Surgical treatment is not normally given in this period. Prisms or occlusion are given temporarily until the condition is stabilized.

9 The general principles of strabismus surgery apply to surgery in paresis, except that recession of the contracted ipsilateral antagonist will be of more value than resection of the paretic muscle. In complete paralysis or severe paralysis a muscle transplantation operation may restore movement in the paretic direction of gaze.

10 Post-operative diplopia may require prisms or occlusion. Horizontal diplopia can often be ignored particularly if one image is degraded, optically or by hypnotic suggestion. Vertical diplopia is more difficult to ignore and in extreme cases scleral contact lenses may be used to provide total occlusion, except for the monocular field of the affected eye which should be left available for safety reasons (see also 4.3).

8.10   Restrictive paresis (synonym: mechanical paresis)

Incomitancy can occur where a muscle is tethered or a systemic disease reduces the elasticity of one or more muscles. An increase of 5 mm in intra-ocular tension when the eye is moved towards the position of restriction compared with the opposite direction, is diagnostic of a mechanical restriction. A hand-held non-contact or pen-type tonometer is ideal for this measurement. The Hess plot may show a restriction of movement in both the main paretic direction and also the opposite direction, though to a lesser extent. The tightly contracted or fibrosed muscle may slip sideways across the globe, away from the normal muscle position, resulting in a sudden up-shoot or down-shoot during a horizontal motility movement because it cannot relax. Restrictions may also be caused by orbital adhesions, due to injury, infection or surgery. An orbital tumour may restrict motility. Sequelae are limited to overaction of the contralateral synergist only.

The measurement of the angle of paretic strabismus, such as Duane's syndrome, cannot be made by cover test, since the paretic eye is restricted to a greater or lesser extent from taking up fixation when the normally fixing eye is covered. If retinal correspondence is normal, as it usually is, a Maddox rod and prism bar may be placed before the paretic eye to measure the deviation. If both eyes are restricted, as in a bilateral Duane's syndrome, Hirschberg reflex testing should be done, or the Krimsky prism test with prisms split equally in front of each eye.

Restrictive pareses are commonly misdiagnosed as neural paresis. Forced duction testing can be performed following topical anaesthesia by using a cotton-bud stick placed on the conjunctiva to move the eye in the direction of the suspected restriction in movement. Forced duction testing using forceps is carried out as a surgical procedure. In either event the oculocardiac reflex should be remembered – bradycardia, nausea and faintness from pressure on the eye or due to stretching the ocular muscles.

8.11   Duane's syndrome

Duane's retraction syndrome is due to a supranuclear brainstem anomaly. This produces third nerve misdirection in lieu of sixth nerve innervation to the lateral rectus causing co-contraction of the lateral rectus and medial rectus muscles. The result is fibrosis of the lateral rectus. Duane's syndrome may occur as part of an inherited triad, with perceptual deafness, and Klippel-Feil syndrome: bony deformities of the neck, usually with fusion of the vertebrae, and thus limitation of neck movement.

Type A shows limited abduction, slightly limited adduction, widening of the palpebral aperture on attempting abduction and reduced convergence.

Type B — as type A but normal adduction.

Type C — adduction more restricted than abduction, exotropia, head turn to assist adduction (see Fig. 8.5).

Vertical retraction syndrome: combined superior and especially inferior rectus paresis. Some degree of retraction when looking up and out may be seen by looking at the cornea from the side.

The *management* of Duane's syndrome is merely treatment of the neonatal amblyopia and correction of the refractive error. Often stereopsis is present and surgery is only required if an abnormal head position is embarrassing the patient.

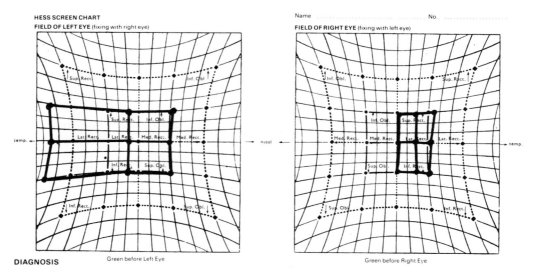

Fig. 8.5 Hess plot: Duane's syndrome, Type C. Right congenital medial rectus restrictive paresis.

8.12   Brown's syndrome

Brown's superior oblique tendon sheath syndrome: congenital restriction or fusion of the superior oblique tendon sheath as it passes through the trochlea (see Fig. 8.6). This can be acquired in injury or in some cases of juvenile rheumatoid arthritis. A Hess plot shows inferior oblique underaction with superior rectus overaction: the contralateral synergist. The superior obliques show an approximately normal plot. In some cases, particularly acquired, repeated attempts to look up and in will produce an audible click, the eye suddenly shooting upwards from a purely horizontal adducted position. The patient may be orthophoric or hypotropic in the affected eye. Diplopia occurs when the affected eye turns in.

The differential diagnosis from inferior oblique paresis is made by the presence of a V pattern (inferior oblique paresis: an A pattern usually), absence of muscle sequelae apart from some overaction of the contralateral synergist: the superior rectus (see Table 8.7).

With a history of recent trauma, the differential diagnosis from orbital floor fracture lies in the absence of elevation of the affected eye in *any* direction upwards: in Brown's syndrome, only elevation in adduction is restricted.

The *management* of Brown's syndrome is tenectomy of the superior oblique muscle in cases of a cosmetically unacceptable head posture, or hypotropia of the affected eye. Otherwise, no treatment is given. Spontaneous recovery may occur: the condition is much less common in adults.

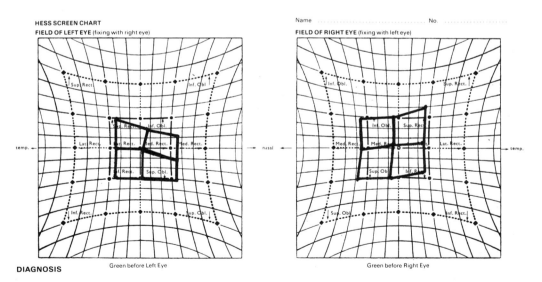

Fig. 8.6 Hess plot. Congenital restrictive LSO paresis: Brown's syndrome, simulating LIO paresis.

Table 8.7 Differential diagnosis: Brown's syndrome/inferior oblique paresis.

	Brown's syndrome	I.O. paresis
A or V pattern	V pattern	A usually
Muscle sequelae		
Overaction of contralateral synergist	Rare	Yes
Contracture of ipsilateral antagonist	No	Yes
Secondary inhibitional paresis of the contralateral antagonist	No	Yes
Vertical deviation	Slight	Marked
Forced duction to test elevation in adduction	Restriction	No restriction
Diplopia on adducting.	Yes, but rare in primary position	Possible, if acquired or becoming decompensated
Symptoms	Pain and discomfort possible with 'click' phenomenon	Rare to complain of pain

8.13   Adherence, fibrosis, strabismus fixus

A congenital adherence of extra-ocular muscles to each other or to fascial tissue runs in families and may also involve the levator muscle. Adhesions may also be acquired due to infection, trauma or surgery.

A congenital inherited fibrosis of some or all extra-ocular muscles causes bilateral ptosis, downward gaze, chin elevation and abnormal convergence movements upon attempted up-gaze or lateral gaze. Strabismus fixus is generally esotropia, but can occur as exotropia and is thought to be caused by secondary fibrosis of muscles contracted as the ipsilateral antagonists of a previous paresis; esotropia would be secondary to a bilateral sixth nerve paresis.

Other anatomical anomalies include variations in the insertion, size (hypertrophy) and path of a muscle, also its total absence.

Adherence and fibrosis will result in restrictions which can be shown by forced duction or tonometry. When the eye is moved maximally in the restricted direction, the intra-ocular tension will be at least 4 mm mercury higher than when in the primary position or the tension of the other eye.

8.14 Traumatic paresis

In traumatic paresis there will be a history of a fall, a fight, or a sports, industrial or road traffic accident (see Figs 8.7 and 8.8). In children, non-accidental injury should be considered: if repeated, the child may avert his gaze or look with sullen watchfulness. Traumatic paresis may be neurogenic (see 8.5) or restrictive. In young children, neurogenic paresis is more likely as 'blow-out' fractures only occur in older children.

A possible examination checklist for suspected non-penetrating eye trauma is as follows:

1 History and symptoms.
2 Visual acuity.
3 External eye examination and slit-lamp: ? hyphaema, ? visible limit to sub-conjunctival haemorrhage.
4 Funduscopy.
5 Is there any pain on eye movement?

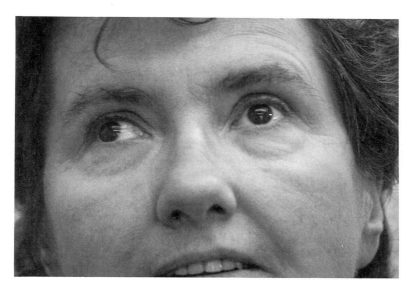

Fig. 8.7 Restrictive bilateral inferior oblique paresis: left inferior oblique paresis shown here. See Fig. 8.8 for Hess plot.

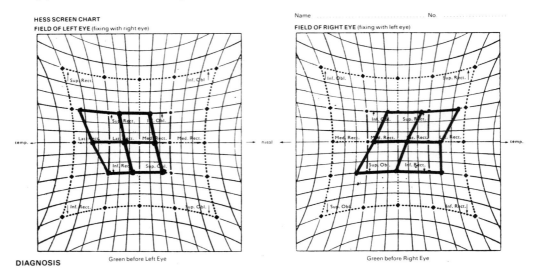

Fig. 8.8 Hess plot. Bilateral inferior oblique restrictive paresis. There is medial rectus underaction and right superior oblique overaction which may be a sequela of a previous left inferior rectus restriction.

6 Is there any pain on palpation? If so, is the pain anterior or retro-bulbar?
7 Visual field examination.
8 Motility, Hess plot, diplopia fields/diplopia matrix.
9 Contrast sensitivity (e.g. A.O./Arden C.S. system).
10 If no abnormality detected, review in 1 week, or sooner if any symptoms appear.

In recent orbital trauma, there may be initial proptosis followed by enophthalmos as the swelling subsides, pain on movement, and a subconjunctival haemorrhage with no visible posterior limit, indicative of an orbital fracture. There may also nose bleeding on the affected side and anaesthesia beneath the lower eyelid. If the orbital trauma was not the main injury there may have been some delay in seeking diagnosis and treatment. A perforating injury may damage any extra-ocular muscle. An orbital fracture may damage the trochlea or the origin of the inferior oblique muscle. Blunt trauma to the orbit may produce a blow-out fracture of the orbital floor, and less commonly the medial wall. The orbital contents are pushed into the crack and the muscles or adjacent tissues are trapped.

A Hess plot will show up-gaze restriction of the affected eye and gross overaction of the other eye in up-gaze (see Fig. 8.9). Blow-outs usually have some restriction on depression because of the mechanical restriction of vertical eye movement. The diplopia will be the *reverse* of the neurogenic paretic effect;

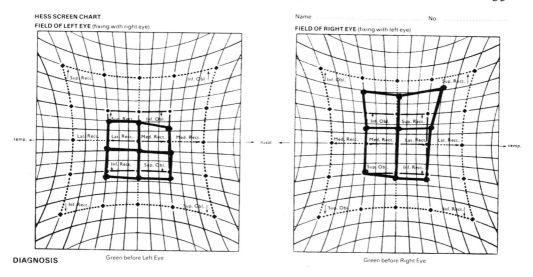

Fig. 8.9 Hess plot: recent left orbital floor fracture — restrictive left inferior oblique paresis. There is overaction of the right eye, both in elevation and depression.

the most peripheral image will belong to the non-paretic eye. Make sure the patient is not further than 50 cm from the Hess screen as the central area may only show a minimal abnormality. The patient will have gross diplopia on looking down on motility testing, but this involves a more peripheral direction of gaze than is available on the Hess screen. The *management* is to review spontaneous improvement at 1 or 2 weeks and then to operate to correct the fracture and to release the trapped tissues.

8.15   Thyroid eye disease (Grave's ophthalmopathy)

Hyperthyroidism usually causes bilateral lid lag (disthyroid myopathy) and lid retraction due to sympathetic stimulation of Müller's muscle. A small proportion have severe changes including gross swelling of the extra-ocular muscles. The muscle action becomes restricted. The swelling also causes exophthalmos and thus exposure keratitis. Contraction of the visual fields is a sign of ischaemic optic neuropathy, although there may be signs of venous stasis in the retina. Young women are at risk of hyperthyroidism. The age group is typically 20–45 years. The first effect is lid retraction, then chemosis, proptosis, diplopia and optic neuropathy. The main symptom is diplopia. The inferior rectus and medial rectus are often first affected. Prisms may be required; as the condition may vary Fresnel press-on prisms are useful. Surgery for diplopia is normally delayed for 2–3 years. Thyroiditis, hypothyroidism and purely ocular Grave's disease also cause related effects. Convergence insufficiency occurs and will require treatment, (see 6.16).

In time, the restricted muscles start to fibrose. Retraction on down-gaze may occur and proptosis on up-gaze. Treatment of hyperthyroidism may result in a patient who is euthyroid or hypothyroid but who may still exhibit the symptoms and signs of thyroid eye disease.

8.16   Myogenic paresis

A direct lesion of an extra-ocular muscle can cause myogenic paresis. Thyroid eye disease begins by muscle swelling (myogenic) but later fibrosis produces a restrictive paresis.

The commonest myogenic paresis is *myasthenia gravis*, which may be general or ocular. Either type presents with ptosis especially when tired, and diplopia then occurs in the majority of cases. This may be provoked by repeated motility testing or Hess testing. Ptosis may be unilateral and may alternate from one eye to the other. Speech and breathing difficulties may occur. The diagnosis is confirmed by intravenous injection of Tensilon (edrophonium chloride) when a rapid improvement in ptosis and diplopia is seen.

Orbital myositis — transient inflammation of a muscle can be due to systemic lupus erythematosis, polyarteritis nodosa and other collagen diseases, or local infection. Often a single muscle is swollen, weakened and unable to relax (with a 'butterfly' facial rash and often alopecia) causing a restrictive effect.

Ocular myopathy is a familial chronic progressive ophthalmoplegia beginning in early adulthood with ptosis often associated with primary retinal pigmentary degeneration. Ptosis-prop contact lenses may be helpful, or a spectacle 'gallery'.

CHAPTER 9

Nystagmus, Irregular Eye Movements, Internuclear and Supranuclear Binocular Anomalies

9.1 Introduction

This chapter covers physiological forms of nystagmus (9.1) and pathological nystagmus — congenital motor (9.2) sensory (9.3) and latent (9.4). Acquired nystagmus is discussed (9.5 to 9.7) and treatment (9.8). Irregular oscillations are mentioned (9.9) and finally internuclear (9.10) and supranuclear binocular anomalies. Nystagmus is recorded as horizontal, vertical or rotary, as pendular or jerky and in which positions of gaze it is present. Nystagmus is a regular binocular oscillation which may be equal (pendular) or unequal (jerky). It occurs physiologically with an optokinetic stimulus, as when looking out of a train window, and in some patients during motility testing (end position nystagmus). This should not be confused with the signs of internuclear ophthalmoplegia. Optokinetic nystagmus has a slow phase following the target and a quick recovery phase. End positional nystagmus has a fast phase in the direction of gaze. Physiological nystagmus can also be produced by vestibular stimulation either by rotating the patient or by pouring hot or cold water in the ear of the supine patient. This causes the fast and slow phase respectively towards that ear (see Fig. 9.1). The mnemonic for 'Cold − Opposite, Warm − Same side' is

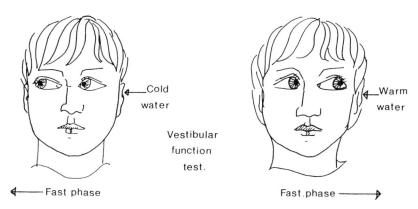

Cold water — Vestibular function test. — Warm water

Fast phase ←   Fast phase →

Fig. 9.1 Vestibular reflex testing.

COWS. Some patients can produce nystagmus voluntarily, while in deepening anaesthesia slow tonic eye movements occur from side to side, sometimes unsynchronized, reducing to stability in the primary position as surgical anaesthesia is reached. In sleep the eyes are stationary or perform slow pendular swings lasting half a second each. REM (rapid eye movement) occurs in sleep in clusters for 20 minutes every 90 minutes (Gay *et al.*, 1974). These symmetrical eye movements are associated with raised temperature, shallow and faster breathing resulting in an increase in pulse rate, other physiological changes and dreaming particularly prior to waking.

A full description of nystagmus and other abnormalities of conjugate eye movement can be found in standard texts (Duke-Elder, 1971; Gay *et al.*, 1974).

9.2   Infantile (pathological) nystagmus (synonym: congenital nystagmus)

The amplitude and speed of infantile nystagmus will be least or absent in the null position which is often in the right field of gaze. To the left of the null position the fast phase will be to the left and to the right on right gaze. A head position may be adopted to bring the null position central, when acuity would improve to 6/24 or better. This use of the null position can produce suppression of the non-dominant eye and hence nystagmus blockage esotropia. Convergence may also reduce the nystagmus. Near visual acuity is important for assessing educational difficulty. The acuity otherwise may be as low as 6/60. Congenital nystagmus does not produce oscillopsia. The nystagmus is horizontal in all fields of gaze.

9.3   Sensory nystagmus

The cone deficiency syndrome may include nystagmus, as may ocular albinism and optic nerve disease or hypoplasia — look for visual field abnormalities. Congenital cataracts, buphthalmos and bilateral corneal opacities may also produce a sensory nystagmus. It is differentiated from infantile nystagmus by the presence of ocular abnormalities, as opposed to a presumed failure of optokinetic control with apparently healthy eyes. In sensory nystagmus the acuity remains unchanged by convergence or direction of gaze. Acuity will be determined by the sensory anomaly.

9.4   Latent nystagmus

In latent nystagmus, when one eye is occluded both eyes show horizontal jerky nystagmus. The fast phase is towards the uncovered eye. The nystagmus may increase on abduction and in this direction it will become manifest even without occlusion. Latent nystagmus can occur in strabismus despite sensory adaptations. To measure acuity in this condition a fogging lens of around +7.00 DS more than the refraction should be used to avoid reduction in VA caused by nystagmus. The differential diagnosis includes irregular nystagmoid movements sometimes found when an amblyopic eye is attempting to fixate.

9.5   Acquired vestibular nystagmus

Here, patients complain of oscillopsia and vertigo. The lesion is in the middle ear, the eighth nerve or its nucleus. It produces a horizontal jerky nystagmus often with a rotary element. Often the nystagmus and symptoms are of short duration as opposed to a central nystagmus where the lesion occurs in the brain stem and the nystagmus is of long duration.

9.6   Gaze paretic nystagmus

Nystagmus can occur when an attempt is made to look in the direction limited by a gaze paresis (see 9.11). The nystagmus is horizontal for lesions in the temporal part of the pons and vertical for segmental mesencephalic damage. It may be found in disseminated sclerosis, encephalitis and certain types of systemic medication, where elevation of the eyes may produce a jerky vertical nystagmus.

A gaze nystagmus occurs in internuclear ophthalmoplegia (see 9.10) on the opposite side to the gaze paresis due to a supranuclear paresis of the medical rectus muscle. This rapid nystagmus increases in amplitude the further the eyes are moved from the primary position. The patient is not normally aware of the nystagmus.

9.7   Rare forms of nystagmus

Positional nystagmus is stimulated by changes in head position and may be due to labyrinthine or central lesions. *Fixation nystagmus* is the result of defective central vision with an abortive attempt to maintain central fixation. *Miner's nystagmus* is pendular and may be due to selection of parafoveal fixation in mesopic conditions. *Vertical nystagmus* may be congenital due to disease or some types of drug addiction, and the fast phase may be up or down (upbeat or downbeat nystagmus). *Upbeat nystagmus* may be due to antihistamine, barbiturates, demyelinating disease or other lesions of the posterior fossa. It can also be due to the limitation of upward gaze in old age, on elevation of the eyes.

Periodically alternating nystagmus has a fast beat to one side for 5 minutes, briefly pauses and then beats to the other side. *Monocular nystagmus* can occur independently or with an internuclear ophthalmoplegia. *See-saw nystagmus* is a pendular movement with intorsion of the upward moving eye and can occur in association with bitemporal hemianopia. In *retraction nystagmus* each oscillation is accompanied by a rapid retraction of both eyes into the orbits with a slow return. *Dissociated nystagmus* describes any nystagmus which shows inter-eye differences in direction or amplitude of movement. It may also accompany *spasmus nutans*: head nodding or shaking, abnormal head position and fine rapid nystagmus. Spasmus mutans usually has an onset in the first 2 years of life and disappears without treatment after a further year. It may however be due to a chiasmal neoplasm.

9.8   Management of nystagmus

Infantile nystagmus and latent nystagmus associated with strabismus will require correction of any significant refractive error: soft contact lenses may produce a better acuity than spectacles but should include correction of astigmatism over 1 dioptre. Hard contact lenses may be difficult to fit without excessive movement of the lens on the eye. Scleral contact lenses should also be considered. Amblyopia should be treated, and surgery for any significant non-accommodative element appears best performed before 24 months old. The surgeon will also consider any abnormal head posture and associated vertical deviation. Convergence excess may be helped with miotics in the short term, bifocal contact lenses or varifocal spectacle lenses in the long term. Equal Fresnel prisms up to 20^Δ may be prescribed base-in one eye and base-out the other with the bases in the direction of a face turn to allow the eyes to utilize the 'null position' while reducing the face turn. The 'null position' is the position of gaze, or of convergence, or both, in which the nystagmus movement is least.

Prisms base-out may be prescribed to utilize the reduction in nystagmus found in convergence. The prism strength is best assessed by its effect on visual acuity and a further assessment made after 3−4 minutes to allow for any prism adaptation. Symmetrical prisms and converging prisms may be combined, again checking the effect on acuity.

Auditory feedback can be used so that patients can aurally monitor their nystagmus and learn to reduce its amplitude (Abadi *et al.*, 1980). The technique is to reflect a spectacle-mounted infra-red light source on to a photocell. The photocell response to the varying light intensity is converted into an audio signal heard by the patient in a hearing aid.

9.9   Ocular irregular oscillations

Dysmetria, flutter and opsoclonus form a spectrum of worsening saccadic control. They may occur in that sequence, or simultaneously, in cerebellar disease.

Oculomotor dysmetria is a consistent binocular overshoot seen on motility testing or on changing fixation from one object to another, often only in one direction. It is due to a lesion of the cerebellum which would normally arrest saccadic movements and maintain fixation.

Ocular flutter also occurs in cerebellar disease and consists of several binocular trembling eye movements when fixation is maintained for a few seconds. Visual acuity drops during these brief episodes.

Opsoclonus is an irregular binocular nystagmoid movement, normally horizontal but may also be rotary or vertical occurring in brief groups of decreasing saccades and stimulated by changes in fixation. It occurs in transient viral encephalitis but also with poliomyelitis and neoplasms.

Ocular myoclonus or 'lightning eye movements' are similar to opsoclonus but are continuous and may continue in sleep. It is associated with gross brainstem pathology, e.g. encephalitis. It may be associated with more general jerking of skeletal muscles: infantile polymyoclonia.

Cogwheel eye movements are seen physiologically in the neonate as an early stage in the development of the fixation reflex. In following a moving object, the eyes make a series of short jumps. Within a few weeks a smooth pursuit movement takes over. In posterior cerebral trauma, encephalitis and homonymous hemianopia, unilateral cog-wheel eye movements occur on attempted pursuit of a target towards the side of the lesion (away from the hemianopia). The lesion would generally be an extensive cerebral infarct or neoplasm, involving the extrapyramidal system and thus muscle tone.

Ocular bobbing describes repeated downward movements of both eyes with a reduction of other eye movements associated with large-scale cerebral haemmorhage.

9.10 Internuclear ophthalmoplegia

Lesions of the *medial longitudinal fasciculus (MLF)* (the nerve pathway which connects the cranial nerve nuclei) produce a characteristic sequence of gradual loss of eye movement. In order, the voluntary, fixation, then pursuit and vestibular eye movement systems are lost. Version (horizontal gaze) movements are controlled by the right and left *paramedian pontine reticular formation* (PPRF) adjacent to the sixth nerve nuclei. The PPRF is the final common pathway for all types of conjugate eye movement.

A *posterior internuclear lesion* in the general area around the sixth nerve nucleus, the PPRF and the MLF will produce a lateral rectus paresis. This is on the same side as the lesion, during binocular motility testing. The lateral rectus paresis does *not* occur during monocular motility. The more common *anterior internuclear lesion* cutting fibres from one third nerve nucleus to the MLF will cause medial rectus paresis on the side of the lesion during motility testing. However, there is *retention* of medial rectus function for convergence. In the early stages, the medial rectus underaction will be better seen by repeated horizontal saccadic testing rather than motility. The affected eye will jerkily undershoot (dysmetria) in adduction while the other eye will simultaneously overshoot in abduction. There will be jerky horizontal nystagmus of one or both eyes when looking in the opposite direction to the paresis.

Internuclear ophthalmoplegia may be unilateral in vascular disease or bilateral in disseminated sclerosis. If bilateral it is unlikely to be symmetrical. A haemorrhage in this area may be secondary to an intracranial space-occupying lesion situated elsewhere. The original symptom may be intermittent diplopia, i.e. in the paretic direction of gaze. The nystagmus may persist after treatment of the cause.

9.11   Supranuclear binocular anomalies

Both normal and abnormal reflex binocular eye movements (i.e. excluding voluntary control) are provided by a combination of conditioned and unconditioned reflexes. Eye movements due to sensory input are mediated by the psycho-optical reflex centres in Brodmann's areas 18 and 19: the fixation and refixation reflexes, the pursuit and the fusional reflexes. It is a conditioned reflex of the fusional system which converts normal binocular vision into concomitant strabismus, with its motor and sensory adaptations.

From areas 18 and 19, stimuli are sent via the MLF to the centres for lateral eye movements (the PPRF − see 9.10 above) and the vertical, convergence and (presumed) divergence centres. (The existence of the divergence centre is postulated from the clinical abnormalities which occur. There is no anatomical evidence for its location.) Other stimuli are brought here from the vestibular system and the frontal voluntary eye movement centres in Brodmann's area 8 (on each side).

Frontal area 8 lesions if merely irritative stimulate unwanted 'voluntary' innervation to produce a conjugate movement of the eyes to the same side as the lesion. This is one form of 'oculogyric crisis', see below. If the lesion becomes destructive the eyes then deviate to the opposite side to the lesion but saccadic movements in that direction are lost; this is a *gaze paresis* (to the same side as the lesion). Often, nystagmus occurs on attempted gaze to the affected side: *gaze-paretic nystagmus*. The pursuit (motility) and vestibular systems are not affected. The right area 8 controls horizontal conjugate gaze to the left, and vice versa. The causes of a gaze paresis include thrombosis, encephalitis and haemorrhage (e.g. due to trauma). The diagnosis of a gaze paresis is aided by the '*dolls head test*' (see 5.10). The *management* of a gaze paresis after referral, and treatment of the immediate cause would include prisms given with their bases in the same direction before each eye.

In congenital (familial) saccadic paralysis (*oculomotor apraxia*) where there is a total absence of saccadic refixation horizontally, a change of fixation is achieved by a head thrust to the side, closure of the eyes and re-opening to allow the vestibular reflex to pull the eyes back onto the desired fixation target. Lesions of the horizontal gaze centre in the PPRF (see 9.10) produce a same-sided gaze paresis for all types of eye movement: pursuit, saccadic and vestibular.

Lesions of the pursuit system are usually due to large areas of parietal or occipital infarction or a neoplasm producing cog-wheel pursuit (see 9.10). Jerky motility movements in old age may be related to this type of lesion but also to extrapyramidal damage, as in Parkinsonism.

Disorders of conjugate vertical gaze are seen as *oculogyric crises* where the eyes move upwards and less commonly laterally or downwards (see Fig. 9.2). This is often associated with post-encephalitic Parkinsonism. Vertical saccades are mediated by both right and left areas 8. The lesion is in the occipital and descending pathways, causing a loss of the fixation reflex. Oculogyric crises may occur in brain-damaged children, but can be learned as a trick by schoolchildren.

In *Parinaud's syndrome* vertical saccades are lost initially, followed by a complete vertical gaze paresis. Occasionally congenital, the cause is usually due to haemorrhage or neoplasm anterior to the corpora quadrigemina.

Parinaud also described *convergence paralysis* with retention of all other monocular and binocular eye movements. The onset is sudden, on attempted convergence both eyes lose fixation together. For distance fixation, prism base-out immediately produces diplopia. The treatment is of the cerebral lesion e.g. disseminated sclerosis. Later, occlusion may be necessary. *Convergence spasm* may occur in irritative lesions, e.g. meningitis.

Divergence paralysis appears as a concomitant esotropia with diplopia for distance vision, but with an absence of ocular muscle paresis or gaze paresis. There is normal binocular vision for near vision with full convergence and

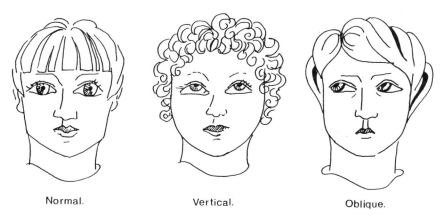

Normal.   Vertical.   Oblique.

Fig. 9.2 Oculogyric crisis types.

accommodation. There would be a history which would include symptoms of cerebral disease such as fits, meningism or pyrexia.

Dissociated vertical deviation (see 7.23) appears to be caused by a lesion of the vertical conjugate gaze centres in the upper mid-brain area.

Double elevator paresis is a unilateral paresis of the inferior oblique and superior rectus muscles of the same eye, (see 8.9). When the unaffected eye fixates, the paretic eye deviates downwards. When the paretic eye fixates the sound eye elevates. Bell's phenomenon (upward movement of both eyes on attempted lid closure) is usually lost. Vertical optokinetic nystagmus and vestibular induced vertical eye movements are retained. The lesion may be an occlusion of the small blood vessels in the vertical gaze centres.

A skew deviation is a temporary vertical 'divergence'. One eye is elevated and the other is depressed. It may be unilateral, but if bilateral, the eyes may reverse the divergence on looking from one side to the other, and thus show incomitancy. In this case, a superior or inferior oblique paresis may be mistakenly diagnosed. There is usually a sudden onset with vertical diplopia. The cause may be brainstem or cerebellar disease.

CHAPTER 10

Professional Qualifying Examination Technique

10.1   Introduction

The professional qualifying examination of the British College of Optometrists is currently (1990) under review. The College is looking at new formats for this examination. One alternative format might include a written paper setting out a patient's history and symptoms. The candidate would indicate which procedures should be investigated in such a patient (e.g. cover test), and which would be contra-indicated (e.g. atropine cycloplegia in an intermittent squint).The details requested would then be revealed and the candidate would then suggest a line of management. For practical skills a series of brief practical examinations on patients, or interpretation of photographs of abnormal conditions, would cover specific points like motility, fixation, convergence, sensory status in squint.

The general content of the examination is likely to remain unchanged. The current examination format has been adopted for discussion here. The candidate should refer to the current syllabus and the guidelines which are readily available from the College. For the (current) P.Q.E. section on anomalies of binocular vision there are two examiners, both optometrists; some examiners have a qualification from the British Orthoptic Council in addition to an optometric qualification. The examiners include university staff and optometrists in hospital or general practice. The examiners will have some postgraduate qualification and experience in teaching undergraduates and/or pre-registration students. They will have experience in clinics or practices with a substantial proportion of patients with anomalies of binocular vision.

10.2   Practice visits

The College arranges practice visits for pre-registration accreditation. A training grant is available to approved practices. When visiting a practice, it is the duty of the college visitor to assist both the supervisor and the trainee in fulfilling the requirements of the pre-registration year. The college visitor will also give advice relating to the professional qualifying examination.

10.3 Oral section

The present Anomalies of Binocular Vision examination is divided into 30 minutes oral and 30 minutes practical, with a different examiner for each. The examiners confer and agree whether a candidate is 'fit to practise' or not. The fundamental consideration is the safety of the public.

Developmental aspects

In the oral, the examiner will be guided by the syllabus and may begin by asking about the development of normal binocular vision. The abnormal cannot be distinguished unless the normal is known. Questions may be asked about the presence at birth of visual and optomotor reflexes: the vestibular (gravitational) system and the proprioceptive neck reflex. The convergence reflex at 3 months should be known, and stereopsis at 4–6 months, active accommodation by 6 months, fixation disparity by 10 months and the maturation of the binocular reflexes at 8 years. Visual acuity development is important, particularly now the Teller and Keeler acuity systems are available for routine use. The examiner may expect knowledge of different methods of obtaining clinical information, for example, dynamic retinoscopy to assess accommodation in young children; or of different stereopsis tests such as the Lang, TNO, Randot, Frisby, Titmus and Mallett. Visual acuity assessments by Catford nystagmus drum and 'hundreds and thousands' are becoming outdated. The Kay test, Sheridan Gardner and Fookes tests, both individual and linearly arranged symbols and the disadvantages of purely silhouette test types should be known. A difference in linear and single letter acuity is a feature of normal visual development. It is abnormal if it persists after 4 years or if marked under this age – greater than 1 or 2 lines on the chart. The half-life of a medical 'fact' is said to be 7 years so bear this in mind – a clear but not dogmatic answer is required.

Causes and classification of binocular vision anomalies

The examiner will want to know if the candidate understands the relationship between accommodation and convergence. AC/A defects cause accommodative squint and convergence excess – phoria or tropia. The AC/A ratio and the refractive error can be used in the management of deviations. The differential diagnosis of the various types of amblyopia is important, or inappropriate management results, for example the orthoptic treatment of a toxic or hysterical amblyopia. The syllabus includes aniseikonia but unless the candidate mentions this topic it is unlikely to arise. Winn *et al.* (1988), suggest that aniseikonia can be corrected by contact lenses in both axial and refractive ametropia.

Investigation and management

The candidate will be expected to describe measurements of the sensory status in squint and heterophoria, the assessment of compensation in heterophoria and monocular fixation patterns in amblyopia. Motility and Hess plot interpretation are likely questions. The diagnostic directions of gaze for the extra-ocular muscles are important, particularly if you have already completed the practical examination and had difficulty with muscle over- or underactions. The examiner may ask about head tilting or turning in paresis (see 5.1). In the management of heterophoria, heterotropia or amblyopia you may be asked how you would manage a general condition: 'How do you treat accommodative squint ... divergence excess ... convergence insufficiency?'. Sometimes the clinical details may be given, but not the technical name of the condition. Usually, the use of a pencil and paper in front of an examiner helps communication. It is best to provide your own materials.

Asking how to treat a condition often produces signs of anxiety in candidates — there are so many treatments. Quite often candidates plump for some exercises which are then described in detail... it is an orthoptic examination after all. A better approach is to outline the general types of treatment in the order in which they should be given.

1 Treat any underlying general health problem.

2 Correct the refractive error and anisometropic problems — unequal image size, convergence, accommodation and variable prism demand. Soft contact lenses with bilateral residual refractive correction by spectacles may be appropiate, for example, to avoid expensive toric soft lenses, or the frequent change of contact lenses for variations in refraction. Monocular or bilateral aphakia in children will require correcting with bifocal or children's varifocal lenses.

3 Consider exercises — positive relative vergences for exodeviations whether phoria, intermittent tropia or divergence excess tropia. Negative relative vergences for decompensated esophoria. Physiological diplopia convergence for convergence insufficiency. Full-time occlusion for amblyopia initially and, if of school age, part-time later with active use of the amblyopic eye. Transferred after-image for teenagers seeking a job with a high visual standard, plus active exercises. Consider refractive modification; bifocals for convergence excess — there is no risk of loss of accommodation since you are only correcting 3 or 4 dioptres out of a total of 10–15 dioptres. Penalization for amblyopia — with or without a cycloplegic. Negative over-correction for exodeviations and convergence insufficiency. Review management frequently at first and not more than 3-monthly if there is any chance of a major change in the patient's binocular condition.

4   Surgery may be necessary (strictly a *surgical opinion*) where the condition is unlikely to be improved significantly by the measures above and presents a cosmetic or functional (diplopia) problem; but not usually for convergence insufficiency or congenital pareses. Marked exophoria responds well to surgery but also to most other forms of treatment.

5   Hypnosis is used to treat post-operative diplopia where the patient has diplopia phobia, and also for the treatment of amblyopia in conjunction with other methods.

6   Finally, the cure for all orthoptic problems, occlusion. This may be given by Fablon or Contact film applied to the back surface of a spectacle lens, or Blenderm film (even more occluding) or a Chavasse or frosted lens. To occlude, a soft contact lens must have an opaque (black) pupil and also an opaque iris colour, otherwise a negative scotoma dances about in front of the patient, varying with pupil size. A scleral lens should be given a clear area to allow vision in the monocular field of vision − this cannot produce diplopia.

No treatment should be given without a thorough check for neurological disorders, repeated 3-monthly: pupil reflexes, monocular accommodation, visual fields, motility, saccadic eye movements, and vergence anomalies, signs of vestibular defects, and a check on the type of amblyopia present (by using a 2.0 ND filter). The management of binocular vision anomalies includes advice about the familial nature of these disorders.

Prognosis and referral

Candidates may be asked, often in the course of a line of questions on investigation and management, to suggest criteria for referral for a medical or surgical opinion. The criteria for a good response to orthoptic or refractive treatment should be known (e.g. superficial rather than deeply ingrained sensory adaptations to a deviation), and indications that any treatment is contra-indicated or likely to be unsuccessful. Functional (not organic) amblyopia generally responds to treatment, but this may take some years if the management is delayed. Decompensated heterophoria, convergence insufficiency and anomalies with a refractive or accommodative element also respond well. Non-accommodative or partially accommodative squints with a residual deviation over $15^{\Delta} - 20^{\Delta}$ may need surgery. The limit of esotropia noticed by parents is 20^{Δ} (until they get more experienced), and about 15^{Δ} for exotropia. About half of exotropias are intermittent and may respond to non-surgical treatment.

Intracranial space-occupying lesions can produce ocular paresis which may first present as a decompensated heterophoria, though with diplopia on extreme eye movement; 80% of brain tumours produce diplopia and have a gradual onset. Aneurysms may show a gradual onset of signs and symptoms unless they start to bleed. Haemorrhages produce sudden onset of diplopia and other symptoms and signs — a stiff neck is typical of a sub-arachnoid haemorrhage. All intracranial space-occupying lesions require referral, but haemorrhages require immediate referral to a district general hospital or neurosurgical unit — the general practitioner should be contacted by phone — the surgery can always use a telephone pager (bleep) if the doctor is not at the surgery. (Their terms of service are to provide 24-hour cover every day of the year.) If the doctor is on a call and a delay is expected before telephoning back, the patient should be sent directly to the hospital with an explanatory letter addressed to the casualty officer. A copy letter should be sent to the GP. A telephone call should be made to the casualty department before sending the patient. Paresis associated with temporal arteritis is also urgent and should be referred to the consultant physician during clinic hours, otherwise to casualty. Referral for a gradual onset diplopia can be made by letter, plus phone call to the GP; brain tumours may be fatal but are not so urgent. The patient should be seen within 24 hours by the GP. In fact, most brain tumours picked up in general optometric practice tend to have a good prognosis, since they are at an earlier stage than those presenting directly to general practitioners.

The referral letter should state the vision and visual acuity, cycloplegic refraction, the angle of the deviation with and without refractive correction and motility. Include details of monocular fixation and binocular sensory status. A copy of the Hess screen chart should be sent where an incomitancy is present. The letter should state the name of the orthoptic anomaly: 'Mr X appears to have...', and the reason for referral e.g. further investigation or recent change in the patient's eyes. By using the word 'appears', the name of the suspected condition can be given to the GP (which is what the GP wants), without the commitment of a conclusive diagnosis, or of excluding the possibility of some additional condition being present.

10.4 The practical examination

The practical examination lasts 30 minutes of which 20 minutes are given for the first patient and 10 minutes for cover test and motility for the second patient. Candidates should bring an occluder, non-focussed pen torch and an ophthalmoscope. Other equipment will be provided at the examination centre. You should ask for equipment if necessary, e.g. a stereopsis test.

The examination record sheet gives the name, age, occupation and current refractive correction of the patient. The correction should be assumed to be optimal for the patient. If the correction includes prisms or has been refractively modified the candidate will generally be told about this. The usual response of patients on being examined is to remove their glasses. This should be resisted as it may alter the binocular status. In fact one examiner is likely to watch part or all of the practical examination because of the variability in patient's responses as they fatigue over the day. There are no restrictions on the questions which candidates may ask, except that if a patient knows he has a named condition such as Duane's syndrome, he will be asked not to divulge this information. In obtaining the history (including family history) and symptoms, the candidate should particularly ask about the age of onset and the current management. Ask about hospital treatment, diplopia and occupational visual problems. Older patients will generally have fewer symptoms and are less likely to be having active therapy. Acute conditions are not likely in an examination but beware the patient who was first seen at the eye clinic recently. The management in this case may not have been finalized. The practical examination of the patient is best made briefly at first, as one would in practice, and then repeated making measurements.

Acuity and cover test

The linear acuity should be taken for each eye. Later the single letter acuity could be taken by holding the examination record sheet so as to cover all but a vertical column of letters on the acuity chart. Next the cover test is performed on the smallest letter which is easily seen by the amblyopic eye, or a spotlight if below 6/18. The B.C.O. Guidelines allow either an estimate or measurement of the deviation, so estimate on the first occasion and measure with a prism bar on repeating the investigation. By asking the patient to make a fixation movement from side to side binocularly from one end of a 6/12 line to the other, an eye movement of 2^Δ can be seen (for a 12 cm line at 6 m). This can be compared with the cover test result. A movement from one side of the chart to the other would approximate 6^Δ. Watch the upper lids — any movement of one lid on cover testing may indicate a vertical component to the deviation. For a phoria, record the speed of the recovery movement as a guide to compensation.

After the distance cover test, tilt the patient's head down and then up, and do the cover test in both positions. An A or V pattern should be easily seen — if none, record 'no A/V pattern'. The near vision cover test should be on a small 'budgie stick' letter at 33 cm. It is very important to have the patient's face adequately illuminated during the cover test. Make a point of adjusting the illumination appropriately.

At this point the glasses may be removed and the cover test measurements repeated. Briefly, but adequately, check the glasses for any prismatic effect.

Motility

Motility should be performed using a non-focussed pen torch so as to equalize retinal image illumination to allow the patient to report diplopia. If a focussed torch is used, aim it at the patient's forehead, not the eyes. Ask if there is any discomfort or inability to move the eyes fully. Watch for diplopia due to metal combination spectacles where only one eye sees through the lens in extreme directions. Check that any diplopia is not due to a high degree of anisometropic spectacle correction. Curve the torch round the patient's eyes as if it were on a perimeter arc, so that equal eye rotations occur. (This is why the Hess screen and chart have pincushion distortion.) If you are at all uncertain about the motility result, do a cover test in the diagnostic directions of gaze (the 'Union Jack' positions, except the vertical bar). Look for a larger cover test movement in one direction of gaze; this will be the paretic direction.

If the patient has diplopia, find out which eye has the outermost (most peripheral) image. If the diplopia is greatest vertically, the images may be obliquely apart. It is the most peripheral image vertically which relates to the underacting eye, except in recent trauma − not likely in an examination. If the patient reports diplopia in all upward directions, but the images are *horizontally* apart, look for a V pattern exodeviation. Other V and A patterns can be worked out on the same basis.

If there is no diplopia, due to suppression or amblyopia, ask the patient how the images jump (when the cover test is performed in each diagnostic direction of gaze) − the image which jumps to the most peripheral position relates to the paretic eye. You may be asked about head posture during the practical examination − remember the head may be moved to bring the diplopic images *together*, or alternatively to *widen* them to allow the paretic image to be ignored. If you have difficulty deciding between, say, a right superior rectus *underaction* and a left inferior oblique *overaction*, the latter is more common in general, but in an examination the patients are more likely to have underactions; in fact pareses are quite likely. A superior rectus paresis often has an associated slight ptosis. Motility should be performed with glasses worn if there is an accommodative element. Monocular motility may be necessary otherwise.

Any other necessary tests

The next heading on the examination record sheet is 'Any other necessary tests'. This covers the sensory status: a Bagolini lens or Mallett fixation disparity test plus a neutral density filter bar will be required to assess retinal correspondence and suppression in heterotropia. Stereopsis and compensation should be checked in heterophoria. Convergence is then measured using an RAF rule. In amblyopia (and only in amblyopia) check fixation of the affected eye with an ophthalmoscope.

Conclusions and recommendations

'Conclusions and recommendations' ideally require the name (not merely a description) of the anomaly present, the onset age if known or estimated, the cause and an outline of suitable management. For example, '20$^\Delta$ right partially accommodative esotropia with convergence excess, onset probably 3 years, associated with hypermetropia, continue with glasses, check cycloplegic refraction and effect of reading addition. Review in 3 months. Check close relatives'. (This ideal is rarely achieved!)

The second patient will require usually one or two investigations suggested by the examiner, and reported orally. These will usually be a cover test and motility. Remember to incorporate the cover test into the motility test as described above: you will be assessed on technique as well as on making the correct diagnosis.

Although this is a practical section of the examination, the examiner may well ask you, 'How you are getting on?'. This may lead to an extensive oral session. Some candidates seem to prefer this to happen. This is possibly because the candidate feels that an oral allows an evaluation of what the examiner is particularly looking for. It may be felt that an oral gives the candidate a chance to adjust gently his opinion about the diagnosis and management. In general, this situation will rarely work to the candidate's advantage. Every piece of information that the examiner gives the candidate, possibly in a genuine attempt to help, is one less piece of information the candidate is able to offer to the examiner. Also the time allowed for examining the patient is ticking away.

To avoid this situation the examination of the patient should be continuous, including a steady conversation with the patient. If a particular test fails to give a satisfactory result, the candidate should move smoothly on to the next test. Only when the routine has been completed should you then return to repeat the unsatisfactory test. A test which is definitely negative should be so recorded. There is very likely something else in that patient which is of particular interest.

Do not worry about obtaining precise measurements of the squint angle or the depth of ARC; these will vary with the subject's fatigue. The main consideration is fitness to practice and safety. The techniques of examining a patient are more important than exact measurements.

10.5 Pre-registration year experience checklist

* **Procedures**
  Cover test
     horizontal phoria
     vertical phoria
     horizontal tropia
     vertical tropia
     latent nystagmus
  Motility:
     objective
     subjective
     utilizing cover test

Convergence:
  push-up
  push-away — failure to follow
  jump
  rotary prism to 20^{Δ}
Sensory status:
  Bagolini ARC
  Bagolini suppression
  Bagolini NRC
  Mallett ARC
  Mallett: suppression (in squint)
  diplopia
  stereopsis
  simultaneous vision only
Compensation:
  compensated phoria
  decompensated phoria
  over-compensated phoria
Monocular fixation:
  central, steady
  central, unsteady
  eccentric, steady
  eccentric, unsteady
  loss of normal foveal localization

- **Binocular anomalies**
  Fully accommodative esotropia
  Partially accommodative esotropia
  Convergence excess esotropia
  Non-accommodative esotropia
  Basic exotropia
  Divergence excess exotropia
  Elevation in adduction
  Paresis
  Nystagmus
  Gaze paresis
  Duane's syndrome
  Convergence insufficiency
  Convergence insufficiency — with low accommodation
  Other anomalies

- **Hospital orthoptic department visits**
- **Question sessions with other students**

Pre-registration year experience checklist (cont.)

- **Reading**

Cashell G.T.W. and Durran I.M. (1980) *Handbook of Orthoptic Principles*, 4th edn. Churchill Livingstone, London.
Hansen V.C. (1988) *Ocular Motility*. Slack Inc., New Jersey.
Lenk-Schäfer M. (Ed) (1987) *Orthoptic Horizons*, Transaction of the 6th International Orthoptic Congress. Harrogate, Great Britain. British Orthoptic Society, London.
Lyle T.K. and Jackson S. (1967) *Practical Orthoptics in the Treatment of Squint*, 5th edn. H.K. Lewis, London.
Pickwell L.D. (1989) *Anomalies of Binocular Vision*, 2nd edn. Butterworths, London.
von Noorden G.K. (1985) *Burian and von Noorden's Binocular Vision and Ocular Motility*, 3rd edn. C. V. Mosby Co., St. Louis.

- **Journals — for up-to-date information**

Journal of Pediatric Ophthalmology and Strabismus. Slack Inc, New Jersey.
Ophthalmic and Physiological Optics. Butterworths Scientific Ltd, Guildford.
Optometry and Vision Science, Williams and Wilkins, Baltimore.
British Orthoptic Journal. British Orthoptic Society, London.
American Orthoptic Journal. University of Wisconsin Press, Wisconsin.

References and Background Reading

Abadi R.V., Carden D. and Simpson J. (1980) A new treatment for congenital nystagmus. *British Journal Ophthalmology*, **64**, 2−6.

Adelstein A.M. and Scully J. (1967) Epidemiological aspects of squint. *British Medical Journal*, **iii**, 334−8.

Apkarian P.A., Nakayama K. and Tyler C.W. (1981) Binocularity in the visual evoked potential: facilitation, summation and suppression. *Electroencephalography and Clinical Neurophysiology*, **51**, 32−48.

Atkinson J., Braddick O. and French J. (1980) Infant astigmatism: its disappearance with age. *Vision Research*, **20**, 891−3.

Atkinson J., Braddick O., Wattam-Bell J., Durden K., Bobier W. and Pointer J. (1987) Photorefractive screening of infants and effects of refractive correction. *Investigative Ophthalmology Vision Science Suppl.*, **28**, 399.

Awaya S. (1978) Stimulus deprivation amblyopia in humans. In *Strabismus, Proceedings of the 3rd Meeting of the International Strabismological Association*, (Ed. by Reinecker R.D.), pp. 31−44. Grune and Stratton, New York.

Bangeter A. (1955) *Amblyopiebehandlung*, 2nd edn. S. Karger, Basel.

Bielschowsky A. (1938) Disturbances of the vertical muscles of the eyes. *Archives of Ophthalmology*, **20**, 175.

Blakemore C. (1974) Maturation and modification in the developing visual system. In *Handbook of Sensory Physiology*, vol. 8. (Ed. by R. Held, H.W. Liebowitz and H.L. Tauber, pp. 377−436. Springer-Verlag, Berlin, New York.

Brown A.M. and Yamamoto M. (1986) Visual acuity in newborn and preterm infants measured with grating acuity cards. *American Journal of Ophthalmology*, **102**, 245−53.

Calder Gillie J. and Lindsay J. (1969) *Orthoptics, a Discussion of Binocular Anomalies*. Hatton Press, London.

Caloroso E. (1972). After-image transfer: a therapeutic procedure for amblyopia. *American Journal of Optometry*, **49**, 65−69.

Caltrider N. and Jampolsky A. (1983) Overcorrecting minus lens therapy for treatment of intermittent exotropia. *Ophthalmology (Rochester)*, **90**, 1160−5.

Campbell F.W., Hess R.F., Watson P.G. and Banks R. (1978) Preliminary results of a physiologically based treatment for amblyopia. *British Journal of Ophthalmology*, **62**, 748.

Catford G.V. and Wilson A. (1981) Miotics in the treatment of squint: a re-appraisal. *British Orthoptic Journal*, **38**, 17.

Charman W.N. (1989) Letter. *Ophthalmic and Physiological Optics*, **9**, 349.

Chavasse F.B. (1939) *Worth's Squint*, 7th edn. Bailliere, Tindall and Cox, London.

Cooper J. (1988) Review of computerised orthoptics with special regard to convergence insufficiency. *American Journal of Optometry and Physiological Optics*, **65**, 455−463.

Cooper J. and Record C.D. (1986) Suppression and retinal correspondence in intermittent exotropia. *British Journal of Ophthalmology*, **70**, 673−6.

Cüppers C. (1956) *Moderne Schielebehandlung. Klinische Monatsblatter für Augenheilkunde*, **129**, 579.

Dobson V., Schwarz T.L., Sandstrom D.J. and Michell L. (1987) Binocular visual acuity in neonates: the grating card procedure. *Developmental Medicine, Child Neurology*, **29**, 199−206.

Douthwaite W.A., Jenkins T.C.A., Pickwell L.D. and Sheridan M. (1981) Treatment of amblyopia by the rotating grating method. *Ophthalmic and Physiological Optics*, **1**, 97−106.

Duke-Elder S. (1971) *System of Ophthalmology*, vol. VI, *Ocular Motility and Strabismus*. H. Kimpton, London.

Duke-Elder S. (1971) *System of Ophthalmology*, vol. XII, *Neuro-ophthalmology*. H. Kimpton, London.

Earnshaw J.R., Goebels W.F., Griffin R.G. and Meakin W.J. (1957) A single mirror haploscope. *Optician*, **133**, 289.

Edwards K. and Llewellyn R. (Eds) (1988) *Optometry*. Butterworths, London.

Eustis H.S. and Parks M.M. (1989) Acquired monofixation syndrome. *Journal of Paediatric Ophthalmology and Strabismus*, **26**, 169−72.

Friedrich D. and de Decker W. (1987) Prospective study of the development of strabismus during the first 6 months of life. In *Orthoptic Horizons*, Transactions of the 6th Orthoptic Congress, Harrogate (Ed. by M. Lenk-Schäfer).

Fitton M.H. and Jampolsky A. (1964) A case report of spontaneous consecutive esotropia. *American Orthoptic Journal*, **14**, 144.

Gay A.J., Newman N.M., Keltner J.L. and Stroud M.H. (1974) *Eye Movement Disorders*. C.V. Mosby Co, St Louis.

Giles G.H. (1943) *The Practice of Orthoptics*. Hammond, Hammond and Co, London.

Graham P.A. (1974) Epidemiology of strabismus. *British Journal of Ophthalmology*, **58**, 224.

Guibor G.P. (1950) Some uses of ophthalmic prisms. In *Strabismus Ophthalmic Symposium I*, (Ed. by J.H. Allen) p. 299. C.V. Mosby Co, St Louis.

Gwiazda J., Brill S., Mohindra I., and Held R., (1980) Preferential looking acuity in infants of 2 to 58 weeks of age. *American Journal of Optometry and Physiological Optics*. **57**, 428−32.

Hansen V.C. (1988) *Ocular Motility*. Slack Inc, New Jersey.

Heaton J.M. (1968) *The Eye, Phenemenology and Psychology of Function and Disorder*. J.B. Lippincott Co, London.

Helveston E.M. and Ellis S.D. (1983) *Paediatric Ophthalmology Practice*. C.V. Mosby, St Louis.

Hofmann F.B. and Bielschowsky A. (1900) Die Verwertung der Kopfneigung zur Diagnose der Augenmuskel lähmungen aus der Heber und Sendkergruppe. v. *Graefes Archive for Ophthalmology*, **51**, 174.

Hugonnier R. and Hugonnier S. (1969) *Strabismus, Heterophoria, Ocular Motor Paralysis*. C.V. Mosby, St Louis.

Humphriss D. (1962) Refraction by immediate contrast. In *Transactions of the International Ophthalmic Optics Congress 1961*, p. 501−10. Crosby Lockwood & Co, London.

Hurtt J., Rasicovici A. and Windsor C. E. (1972) *Orthoptics and Ocular Motility*. C.V. Mosby Co., St. Louis.

Ingram R.M., Walker C., Wilson J.M., Arnold P.E. and Dally S. (1986) Prediction of amblyopia and squint by means of refraction at age 1 year. *British Journal of Ophthalmology*, **70**, 12.

Jampolsky A.J. (1989) Discussion (of Eustis *et al.*, 1989). *Journal of Paediatric Ophthalmology and Strabismus*, **26**, 173–5.

Jenkins T.C.A., Pickwell L.D. and Yekta A.A. (1989) Criteria for decompensation in binocular vision. *Ophthalmic and Physiological Optics*, **9**, 121–5.

Jennings J.A.M. (1985) Anomalous retinal correspondence – a review. *Ophthalmic and Physiological Optics*, **5**, 537–68.

Lang J. (1982) New stereotests. In *Proceedings of the International Symposium on Strabismus* (Ed. by M.C. Boschi and R. Frosini), p. 177 Florence, Italy, June 21–23, 1982.

Lang, J.I. and Lang T.J. (1988) Eye screening with the Lang stereo test. *American Orthoptic Journal*, **38**, 48–50.

Mallett R.F.J. (1964) The investigation of heterophoria at near and a new fixation disparity technique. *Optician*, **148**, 547–51.

Mallett R.F.J. (1966) A fixation disparity test for distance use. *Optician*, **148**, 1–3.

Mallett R.J.F. (1974) Fixation disparity – its genesis in relation to asthenopia. *Ophthalmic Optician*, **14**, 1159–68.

Mallett R.J.F. (1979) The use of prisms in the treatment of concomitant strabismus. *Ophthalmic Optician*, **19**, 793–8.

McDonald M., Ankrum C., Preston K., Sebris S.L., and Dobson V. (1986) Monocular and binocular acuity estimation in 18 to 36-month-olds acuity card results. *American Journal of Optometry and Physiological Optics*. **63**, 181–6.

Mein J. (1983) The asymmetrical optokinetic response. *British Orthoptic Journal*, **38**, 17.

Mein J. and Harcourt B. (1986) *Diagnosis and Management of Ocular Motility Disorders*. Blackwell Scientific Publications, Oxford.

Mitchell D.E., Freeman R.D., Millodot M. and Haegerstrom G. (1973) Meridional evidence for modification of the human visual system by early visual experience. *Vision Research*, **13**, 535–58.

Mohindra I., Held R., Gwiazda J. and Brill S. (1978) Astigmatism in infants. *Science*, **202**, 329–31.

North R. and Henson D.B. (1981) Adaptation to prism induced heterophoria in subjects with abnormal binocular vision or asthenopia. *American Journal of Optometry and Physiological Optics*, **58(a)**, 746–52.

North R.V., Sethi B. and Owen K. (1990) Prism adaptation and viewing distance. *Ophthalmic and Physiological Optics*, **10**, in press.

Pickwell L.D. (1989) *Binocular Vision Anomalies*. Butterworths, London.

Reinecker R.D. (1978) *Strabismus, Proceedings of the 3rd Meeting of the International Strabismological Association*. Grune and Stratton, New York

Reinecker R.D. (1982) *Strabismus II, Proceedings of the 4th Meeting of the International Strabismological Association*. Grune and Stratton, New York.

Revell, M.J. (1970) *Strabismus, a History of Orthoptic Techniques*. Barry and Jenkins, London.

Rutstein R.P., Daum K.M. and Eskridge J.B. (1989) Clinical characteristics of anomalous correspondence. *Optometry and Visual Science*, **66**, 420–5.

Schor C.M. and Ciuffreda K.J. (1983) *Vergence Eye Movements: Basic and Clinical Aspects*. Butterworths, Boston.

Scott A. (1981) Botulinum toxic injection of the eye muscles to correct strabismus. *Transactions of the American Ophthalmological Society*, **79**, 734.

Sheridan M.D. (1969) Vision screening procedures for very young or handicapped children. In *Aspects of Developmental and Paediatric Ophthalmology*. (Ed. by P. Gardiner, R. Mac Keith, and V. Smith, Heinemann Medical Books Ltd, London.

Sondhi N., Archer S.M. and Helveston E.M. (1988) Development of normal ocular alignment. *Journal of Paediatric Ophthalmology and Strabismus*, **25**, 210–1.

Stidwill D.B. (1987) Simulation of squint. *Ophthalmic and Physiological Optics*, **7**, 87.

Thompson C. and Drasdo N. (1988) Clinical experience with preferential looking acuity tests in infants and young children. *Ophthalmic and Physiological Optics*, **8**, 309–21.

von Noorden G.K. (1985) *Burian and von Noorden's Binocular Vision and Ocular Motility*, 3rd edn. C.V. Mosby Co, St Louis.

Walraven (1949) In *Clinical Orthoptics: Diagnosis and Treatment*. (Ed. by M.E. Kramer), p. 349. C.V. Mosby Co, St Louis.

Worth C. (1929) *Squint, its Causes, Pathology and Treatment*. 6th edn. Baillière, Tindall and Cox, London.

Westall C.A. (1981) Physiological background to amblyopia treatment by rotating gratings. *Ophthalmic and Physiological Optics*, **1**, 175–85.

Winn B., Ackerley R.G., Brown C.A., Murray F.K., Prais I. and St. John M.F. (1988) Reduced aniseikonia in axial anisometropia with contact lens correction. *Ophthalmic and Physiological Optics*, **8**, 341–344.

Case Histories

Esophoria

James B. Age 9

Referred for low VA.
R +1.75 DS: 6/6
L +1.75/−1.00 × 10: 6/12.
Distance: 13$^\Delta$ SOP. Near: 11$^\Delta$ SOP. Intermittent decompensation and suppression for distance and near fixation, without and with trial lenses. Stereopsis 60″ TNO. Motility full.

Assessment

This is an example of partially refractive esophoria (see 6.2, 7.5). Given glasses to fully correct the refractive error, evening and weekend occlusion, and anti-amblyopia exercises: fine writing and identifying coloured letters of decreasing size.

10 months later. SOP now compensated for distance and near vision, with glasses. Exercises and occlusion discontinued VA R 6/6 + L 6/6.

3 months later. Glasses discontinued, for review at decreasing intervals.

Comment

The phoria may have decompensated due to fatigue, resulting in facultative/obligatory suppression and amblyopia. The initially good stereopsis indicated that the decompensation was not long-standing, and the prognosis was good — eventual regain of control without glasses.

Andrew E. Age 25

Patient complained of eyestrain at work and home. Glasses worn to improve acuity.

R +0.75/+1.50 × 100: 6/6
L Plano/+0.75 × 105: 6/6
Distance: 10$^\Delta$ SOP (3$^\Delta$ to compensate). Near: 10$^\Delta$ SOP, (3$^\Delta$ to compensate).
Motility full.

Assessment

Decompensated partially refractive esophoria (see 6.2, 7.5).
    Given: R 0.75/+1.50 × 100 = 1.5 prism base-out; L Plano/+0.75 × 105 =
1.5 prism base-out.

Comment

This is the heterophoria equivalent of partially accommodative esotropia. So
surgery would have been an alternative form of management. In that case glasses
might no longer be necessary.

Angela E. Age 25

No symptoms, wears glasses to improve acuity.
R +0.75/+1.50 × 100: 6/6
L −1.00/+1.00 × 105: 6/5
Distance: 7$^\Delta$ SOP (compensated). Near: 4$^\Delta$ SOP (compensated).
    12 years later. Complains of eyestrain at work and home. Distance and near:
10$^\Delta$ SOP (3$^\Delta$ to compensate): acuity R 6/9 L 6/5. Motility: full.

Assessment

Partially refractive esophoria (see 6.2, 7.4).
    Given: R +1.00/+1.5 × 105 = 1.5$^\Delta$ base-out; L Plano/+1.00 × 135 =
1.5$^\Delta$ base-out.

Comment

Note:
1 Reduced acuity in right eye is a sign of suppression and amblyopia. This is
   a response to confusion produced by binocular instability, i.e. intermittent
   decompensation.
2 Compensation was initially achieved by correcting the hypermetropia and by
   providing clear retinal images. Later, prisms were given to help control
   decompensation arising from the anatomical component of the deviation.
3 The symptoms appearing in 1989 were possibly due to stress or fatigue.

Exophoria

Anthony G.A. Age 23

Complained of poor unaided vision in the left eye.
6/5: R +0.25 DS: 6/5
6/12: L +0.50/−1.50 × 5: 6/6.
Distance: 12^Δ L intermittent XOT. Near: 20^Δ XOP, stereopsis 480″. Motility full.

Assessment

Basic exotropia. Given full refractive correction.
   10 years later. L XOT only when tired. Distance: 11^Δ XOP/T. Near: 18^Δ XOP. Stereopsis 480″.

Comment

This case of intermittent L XOT was managed by refractive correction only. Stereopsis remained unchanged. Alternative management would include assessment for prism correction and surgery. The subnormal stereopsis may be due to an inadequate control of the deviation. Alternatively it may not have been capable of improvement with a patient presenting at age 23, with what was probably a congenital intermittent deviation (see 7.15).

Lucy M.A. Age 6

Parents report intermittent R XOT for 13 months, more frequent lately.
R +0.50/+4.00 × 110: 3/9
L +0.50/+4.00 × 80: 3/6
Distance and near: 20^Δ R intermittent XOT (can alternate). Stereo 2000″, with and without refractive correction. Motility full.

Assessment

A basic exodeviation of congenital origin, which decompensated into a manifest deviation around the time of school entry.
   Given full refractive correction.
   3 months later. Distance and near: 20^Δ (variable) R XOP/T. Manifest deviation only noticed when tired. Stereopsis 200″.

Comment

Again only a refractive correction was given. Stereopsis improved from 2000″ to 200″ TNO in 3 months, and further improvement is likely. A failure to improve would indicate the need for additional supportive measures including exercises to improve positive relative vergence, negative refractive modification, prisms or surgery (see 7.15).

Esotropia

George G.H. Age 5

School referral for reduced vision: R 6/9 L 6/9.
R +2.00/+1.00 × 180: 6/9
L +2.00/+1.00 × 170: 6/9
History of strabismus in aunt. Motility: slight LSR underaction. Congenital left ptosis. Stereopsis 100″.

Fixation disparity test gives normal result − no suppression or decompensation. Distance vision 4^Δ SOP. Rx: for review 3/12

10 months later. Cover test: 10^Δ L SOT for distance and near vision. Acuity R 6/6−3 L 6/9−3. Stereopsis: none. Left ptosis more marked − eyelid almost closes when tired. Rx: refractive correction given.

Assessment

Late onset partially accommodative esotropia.

3 months later. Stereopsis 100″. Acuity R 6/9 L 6/9−3.

10 months later. Cover test: distance vision; straight, near vision; 10^Δ L SOT. With reading addition of +2.50, near deviation reduces to 3^Δ SOP (compensated). Given bifocals.

3 months later. Requires 4^Δ base-out each eye to compensate distance and near vision. Given prism bifocals.

2 years later. Patient gets diplopia when tired if not wearing above correction. Distance: 10^Δ L SOP/T, compensated with 2^Δ base-out each eye. Near: 9^Δ L SOP/T through top of glasses, 6^Δ L SOP/T through segment. The diplopia indicates the patient has normal binocular vision when not diplopic − i.e. most of the time. Stereopsis 2000″.

1 year later. Age 10 years. Can manage without glasses unless tired. Stereopsis 200″. Distance: 5^Δ SOP/T without glasses. Near: 6^Δ SOP/T without glasses. The appearance of diplopia when tired protects the patient against unsuspected adverse motor or sensory adaptations.

Comment

This case history documents the gradual failure of binocular vision due to a partially accommodative esophoria with convergence excess, decompensated by increasing ptosis. The management is then described. The increase in ptosis was due to fatigue with the increasing demands put on a school entrant. The patient's father was a medical practitioner and the congenital ptosis was investigated in early childhood. As the child passed the critical age of 8–10 years with good control, the need for supportive measures decreased (see 7.4).

Exotropia

William M. Age 52

Complains of right proptosis. Hyperthyroidism diagnosed. Distance: 4^Δ XOP, compensated. Near: 10^Δ XOP, compensated.

8 years later. Right early cataract reduces acuity to R 6/12 L 6/6 and phoria decompensates when tired, for near vision. Distance: 4^Δ XOP. Near: 16^Δ XOP/T, 1^Δ base-in each eye to compensate. NPC: 30 cm. Accommodation: 2 DS. Stereopsis: 100″. Motility: some limitation in elevation and on right eye abduction. Exophthalmometry R24 L21.

Assessment

Initially myogenic, and later restrictive, paretic intermittent exotropia.

Given: R Plano = 1 prism base-in; L Plano = 1 prism base-in; add + 2.00 = same prisms.

2 years later. Listed for intra-ocular lens implant.

Comment

This patient with hyperthyroidism had proptosis which was produced by oedema of the extra-ocular muscles, particularly the RMR and RLR. In turn this increased the XOP for near vision and decreased the NPC to 30 cm. This would be a static rather than a dynamic effect – failure to converge on a Maddox wing test will result in a reading of around 18^Δ XOP. The problem was made worse by incipient cataract in the same eye and at this point the phoria decompensated intermittently. Prisms were needed to compensate for near vision, and although not required for distance vision, were incorporated in both distance and near elements of a bifocal correction. The patient was able to adapt to the unnecessary prisms for distance fixation, particularly as he had (compensated) XOP for distance vision. The alternative of prism controlled bifocals would have been expensive, difficult to obtain and in fact, disruptive of binocular control when changing from distance to near fixation or vice versa (see 7.20, 7.21, 8.15 and 8.16).

Amblyopia

Sally V.G. Age 7

School referral for reduced vision.
R +9.00/−3.00 × 180: 6/18
L +9.00/−3.00 × 180: 6/18
Distance: 6^Δ XOP. Near: 4^Δ XOP.

Assessment

Congenital refractive amblyopia.
  Given glasses and anti-amblyopia exercises (see 4.13).
  1 year later. Acuities R 6/12 L 6/12. Anti-amblyopia exercises continued: fine writing, recognition of coloured letters of decreasing size, Keeler Projectoscope and Nutt Autodisc pleoptic treatment.
  2 years later. Given contact lenses: acuities R 6/9 L 6/12+. Distance: 6^Δ XOP. near: 4^Δ XOP.

Comment

The treatment of bilateral amblyopia requires correction of the refractive error, aniseikonia and any binocular imbalance which might encourage suppression. Cases of spherical anisometropia or equal refractive error with different astigmatic axes in each eye, are best corrected with contact lenses. Even where the axes are identical, as here, a distortion in retinal images will be reduced by contact lenses. The other adverse effects of anisometropic correction by spectacles should also be noted − induced prismatic effects in version and vergence movements and unequal amounts of convergence and accommodation for each eye. Bilateral amblyopia will generally need active therapy. Pleoptics, the CAM stimulator, and more recently the Mallett IPS unit have been used in these cases. Although normal acuity was not achieved, the patient was able to pass the visual requirement for driving (see 4.13).

Convergence insufficiency

Shiela C.B. Age 15

Complains of diplopia for near vision. Convergence exercises had been given without any improvement. Acuities R 6/6 L 6/6. NPC 50 cm. Distance: 4^Δ XOP, compensated. Motility: full, accommodation 3 DS each eye.

Assessment

Convergence and accommodative insufficiency.
Given: R +0.50/−0.50 × 30 = 3$^\Delta$ base-in; L +0.75/−0.50 × 150 = 3$^\Delta$ base-in; add +2.50 = same prism.

9 years later. NPC is 25 cm with above correction. Given: R +0.50/−0.50 × 30 = 5$^\Delta$ base-in; L +0.75/−0.50 × 150 = 5$^\Delta$ base-in; add +2.50 = same prism.

This prescription was given for clerical work. To use previous Rx for ward duty (nursing). NPC: 55 cm Accommodation: 3 DS.

Comment

Orthoptic exercises to correct convergence insufficiency are usually highly successful. In some cases regression occurs when treatment ceases. Where accommodation is low also, the prognosis for cure is less good. Symptomatic relief may then be appropriate, as here and will be necessary permanently (see 6.17 and 6.19).

Denise A.B. (sister of SCB) age 17

Complains of headaches and diplopia. NPC 50 cm. Accommodation: 2.5 DS (each eye). Motility: full. VA R 6/6. L 6/6 Distance: 1$^\Delta$ SOP. Near: 10$^\Delta$ XOP, compensated.

Trial of Fresnel bifocals and prisms given to investigate possibility of binocular vision at near − impractical to prescribe sufficiently high prisms for normal use.

Assessment

Convergence and accommodative insufficiency.

Given: R +0.75 DS; L +0.75 DS; add +3.00 varifocal with Fablon occlusion on back surface of the left lens. To be worn for near vision only.

2 years later. Can achieve NPC 10 cm with extreme effort, but otherwise 50 cm. Can manage without glasses by holding reading material away, by looking away to rest eyes and by avoiding poor lighting levels.

Comment

As for SCB above.

Paresis

Jane H. Age 60

Complains of sudden recent diplopia and R XOT with right ptosis. Motility: slight further movement to the right only (right eye); left eye − full movement.

Assessment

Third nerve lesion, probably of vascular origin affecting extra-ocular muscles.

Patient saw a consultant neurologist who diagnosed a right third nerve lesion of unknown origin and referred for ophthalmological assessment. Patient's husband occluded the right lens of her glasses to stop diplopia. Exercises were given to converge and diverge binocularly in extreme dextroversion, and also to turn the head to the right slowly while maintaining binocular fixation on an object to the patient's right.

1 month later. Fusion possible in the primary position with 25^{Δ} base-in each eye.

1 month later. Fusion possible in the primary position with 8^{Δ} base-in each eye.

1 month later. Fusion possible in all directions except extreme laevo-version without prisms. Acuity, visual fields, fundi, pupil reflexes were normal.

Comment

Although the cause was unknown, the sudden onset and rapid improvement is consistent with a cerebral vascular accident, i.e. a haemorrhage or thrombosis. Pareses often improve, following treatment of the primary cause if known. The overaction of the ipsilateral antagonist may persist (as a contracture). Appropriate management should minimize this sequela.

Revision Questions

Chapter 1

- At what age is kinetic nystagmus present? (1.1)
- What is the monocular acuity at birth? (1.1)
- How does average refraction change between birth and five years? (1.1)
- At what age can stereopsis be checked in practice? (1.1)
- What are the critical and plastic periods in visual development? (1.2)

Chapter 2

- What is a 'deviation' in orthoptic terminology? (2.1)
- How may an extra-ocular muscle be weakened? (2.2)
- How did Worth grade binocular sensory anomalies? (2.3)
- How does the Opticians Act regulate orthoptics? (2.3)

Chapter 3

- How does a partially accommodative squint occur? (3.2)
- How many systems of eye movement are there? (3.3)
- Fixation disparity may be regarded as (i) a trigger to fusional vergence and (ii) ...? (3.5)
- Symptom-free decompensation of a phoria in children may produce ...? (3.5)

Chapter 4

- What is the difference between diplopia and confusion? (4.1)
- What may facultative suppression become, if untreated? (4.1)
- How does ARC develop? (4.1–4.7)
- How may diplopia be recorded over the binocular field? (4.3)
- What is the most sensitive test for suppression? (4.4)

Chapter 5

- How may an abnormal head posture benefit a paretic patient (5.1)
- What abnormality is associated with the crowding phenomenon (5.5)
- What can be deduced from the speed of recovery from cover test occlusion? (5.6)
- What is the difference between the habitual and total squint angle? (5.6)
- How may ARC invalidate a Hess screen test? (5.12)
- In squint, a Bagolini streak seen through the fixation spotlight by the deviated eye indicates ... (5.14)

Chapter 6

- Failure of the vergence system to maintain inadequate fusion in heterophoria produces ... (6.3)
- The most common cause of such failure is ... (6.3)
- To correct decompensation in heterophoria three techniques may be applied ... (6.9)
- Suppression can be treated by the following four techniques ... (6.10)
- Positive relative vergence may be improved by the following four techniques ... (6.15)
- Convergence insufficiency may be improved by the following four techniques ... (6.15−6.20)

Chapter 7

- The peak onset of fully accommodative squint is between ... and ... years (7.2)
- The management of fully accommodative squint is primarily ... (7.2)
- A convergence excess accommodative squint has a high/low AC/A ratio (typically ...). The primary treatment is ... (7.3)
- Miotics may be used as a temporary alternative, or in addition to ... (7.3)
- Transferred fixation is used to treat ... in partially accommodative squint.
- Divergence excess may be treated by ... lenses, exercises or ... (7.16)

Chapter 8

- Following a recent paresis of the RLR overaction of the ... will occur, followed by ... of the ipsilateral antagonist. ... (8.1−8.7)
- A later effect is secondary inhibited paresis of ... (8.1−8.8)
- The commonest A or V pattern is a ... pattern tropia. (8.1−8.8)

- A complete third nerve paresis will produce failure of the following extra-ocular eye muscles ... and intra-ocular muscles ... and cause the lid to ...
- An example of myogenic paresis is ...

Chapter 9

- Latent nystagmus can be demonstrated by ... (9.4)
- Gaze paresis nystagmus treatment is given to correct the refractive error and reduce the amplitude of movement by ... (9.2−9.8)
- ... exercises may also help to reduce nystagmus (9.2−9.8)
- Oculo-motor dysmetria is seen on motility testing as ... An internuclear lesion between the sixth and seventh nerves will produce ... and nystagmus.

Case histories

Patients 1 and 2 presented like this: patient 1 had reading difficulty and showed 5^Δ SOP for distance and near vision. Patient 2 complained of 'pulling on the eyes' when tired, and had 5^Δ SOP at distance, orthophoric for near fixation.

In each case, what would be the most important part of the investigation? Would a cycloplegic refraction help? What steps would you take to manage these patients?

Short answers are: the full refraction is crucial, any decompensation with the full Rx should be assessed. Patient 1 may need a bifocal correction, patient 2 may require prisms base-out for distance; and though not required for near vision, the patient should readily adapt to the same prism strength. If control worsened, a surgical opinion should be sought. As you reconsider patient 1, do you find section 7.4 to be more appropriate than section 7.6 or vice versa?

Patients 3 and 4, both aged 5, presented with RSOT. Patient 3 had hyper-metropia, but patient 4 was emmetropic. In each case, what do you think would be the most important part of the investigation? Which do you think is the more likely to be incomitant? Which has the better prognosis without surgery? Short answers to these questions are: the most important part of the investigation is cycloplegic refraction and motility. Case 4 may be incomitant, especially if the squint is of recent origin. Case 3 would have the better prognosis without surgery. As you reconsider patient 3, look at sections 7.2 and 7.4, and for patient 4, sections 8.1 and 8.5. Which muscle would you expect to overact if a paresis was present?

Patients 5 and 6 complain of reading difficulty. They are both orthophoric emmetropes in their early twenties. What investigations would you make? Both have a near point of convergence of 25−30 cm, and patient 6 has only 3 dioptres of accommodation. How would you manage these patients? Is incomitancy possible — if so, where might the lesion be found? Short answers to these questions are: investigate cycloplegic refraction and convergence, contrast sensitivity (which will be affected in retro-bulbar neuritis, e.g. disseminated sclerosis), colour vision and visual fields. Management: check that the symptoms are not associated with transient illness. (Note that nasal decongestants can affect accommodation.) Then treat patient 5 with convergence exercises. Patient 6 is less likely to respond to exercises, and may need bifocals and base-in prisms. Review both patients at 1 and 3 months, including a check on motility and visual fields. Incomitancy may account for convergence insufficiency in patient 5, due to a lesion adjacent to the right and left fourth nerve nuclei. A Hess plot would confirm this. Patient 6 is more likely to have a long-standing deficit of accommodation and convergence, which may have become more apparent with a change in occupation or due to stress. In considering these patients, which of sections 6.17—6.23 do you consider more applicable respectively?

Patients 7 and 8 each report momentary horizontal diplopia when recently driving long distances at night. What would be the most serious cause? What would be the most likely? What unusual causes of diplopia might you exclude? Following assessment, patient 7 is diagnosed as having a decompensated basic exophoria. Patient 8 has divergence excess. Give the management protocol in each case, listing treatment in the order in which it should be given. Short answers: the most serious cause of intermittent diplopia would be paresis due to haemorrhage, neoplastic or demyelinating disease. The most likely cause is a congenital concomitant exodeviation, decompensating under adverse conditions. (Decompensation of an old paresis is seen less frequently.) Unusual causes of diplopia include transient astigmatism caused by a chalazion, corneal and lens opacities, macular oedema, the prismatic effects of an anisometropic spectacle correction, or from an excessively mobile hard contact lens, and intermittent lapses of fusion in patients with visual field loss. In considering management, which of sections 7.15—7.21 do you feel are applicable?

Patients 9 and 10 are referred to you, aged 4 years, each with abnormal head positions. What would be the most important aspects of the investigation? In patient 9, reversing the head tilt (to the opposite side) still does not produce any hyperdeviation. What would be the tentative diagnosis? In patient 10, upon straightening the head, horizontal jerk nystagmus occurs. What is the most likely diagnosis? Short answers: the most important aspects of investigation would be motility and reversing the head tilt. Patient 9 is likely to have a congenital orthopaedic torticollis, (but note, both orthopaedic and ocular types can co-exist). Patient 10 is likely to have a congenital nystagmus controlled by the abnormal head position. In considering these patients, which other diagnoses must be excluded? Look at sections 7.9, 8.8, 8.13, 8.15 and 8.16.

Glossary

Abduction: Lateral rotation of one eye from the primary position.

Accidental alternation: An alternating strabismus in which one eye usually fixates. An inappropriate term since most alternating squints do this. See, *essential alternation.*

Adduction: Medial (nasal) rotation of one eye from the primary position.

Agonist: A muscle receiving primary innervation to contract, so as to move the eye into a new direction of gaze.

Alternating deorsumduction: A form of dissociated vertical deviation where either eye deviates downward under cover.

Alternating strabismus: A strabismus with no preference for fixation by either eye, for distance and/or near fixation.

Alternating sursumduction: A form of dissociated vertical deviation where either eye deviates upwards under cover.

Amblyopia: A reduction in visual acuity that is not associated with any visible or refractive abnormality of the eye (see 4.8 for classification of amblyopia types).

Amplitudes: See, *relative vergences*

Angle, alpha: The angle between the approximate optic axis of the eye and the line of sight.

Angle, gamma: The angle between the approximate optic axis of the eye and the fixation axis at the average centre of rotation of the eye.

Angle, kappa: See, *angle, lambda.*

Angle, lambda: The angle between the pupillary axis and the line of sight, measured at the nodal point. (Commonly called 'angle kappa'). It is positive when the visual axis is nasal to the pupillary axis; if large it causes pseudo-exotropia.

Angle, objective: The angle of deviation measured by prism cover test, or by alternately illuminating each tube of a synoptophore and adjusting it until there is no eye movement.

Angle of anomaly: The difference between the objective and subjective strabismus angles in ARC, e.g. when measured with a synoptophore-type instrument.

Angle, primary and secondary: See, *primary deviation, secondary deviation.*

Angle, subjective: The angle of a deviation, measured by asking the patient to move one tube of a synoptophore until the two images appear to be fused.

Anomalous retinal correspondence (ARC, abnormal retinal correspondence): Normally non-corresponding retinal areas of each eye (receiving the same image due to strabismus) acquire a common visual direction under binocular conditions. See, *harmonious ARC*.

Antagonist: The muscle which receives primary innervation to relax when the agonist contracts. The ipsilateral antagonist is on the same eye, and the contralateral antagonist on the opposite eye to the agonist.

Associated phoria: The amount of prism required to align the nonius marks on a fixation disparity test.

Bielschowsky's sign: Depression of the covered eye in alternating sursumduction when a filter is placed before the fixing eye.

Binocular duction measurements: See, *relative vergence*

'Binocular lock': The visual input which is common to both eyes, and thus helps to maintain fusion (see 6.3).

Binocular single vision (BSV): Normal binocular vision. Binocular single vision also occurs in ARC, so BSV should strictly be called 'normal binocular single vision'.

Binocular triplopia: A temporary persistence or re-appearance of pre-operative ARC coupled with post-operative ARC or, if the eyes are straight, NRC.

Blind spot syndrome: Obsolete description for an esotropia of $12-15°$.

Cardinal directions of gaze: The six diagnostic gaze positions used for assessing the presence of incomitancy or paresis.

Concomitant (comitant): A condition where the angle between the visual axes remains constant, in all directions of gaze, for a given fixation distance.

Confusion: The visual disturbance created in a recent strabismus by dissimilar images falling on each fovea and being projected to the same position in visual space.

Conjugate movements: Equal rotation amounts of the two eyes (horizontally, vertically, obliquely or around the visual axes) in the same direction.

Convergence: Medial (nasal) rotation of both eyes, normally to fixate a nearer object.

Convergence excess: A esodeviation which is greater for near vision than for distance fixation.

Convergence insufficiency: A near point of convergence greater than 10 cm, or poorly sustained on repeated testing, or a convergence amplitude of less than 20^{Δ}. Treatment would be given where symptoms were present.

Convergence weakness: An exodeviation greater for near vision than for distance fixation.

Corresponding points: Small retinal areas of each eye sharing the same visual direction.

Decompensation: The loss of control by the vergence eye movement system, over heterophoria. It results in a decompensated phoria, then an intermittent tropia if further control is lost. It can occur when an old paresis becomes grossly incomitant again.

Deviation: In this text, heterophoria or heterotropia (or combinations of both in different directions or distances of gaze). In other texts, the term may be used for heterotropia only, or purely to describe gaze paresis and related defects.

Diplopia: Two images of the same object are seen because they fall on non-corresponding retinal points.

Disjugate movements: Rotation of the two eyes (horizontally, vertically, obliquely or around the visual axes) in opposite directions.

Dissociated phoria: The heterophoria measured under dissociation. See also, *associated phoria*.

Divergence: Lateral (temporal) rotation of both eyes, normally from a position of convergence.

Divergence excess: An exodeviation greater for distance vision than for near fixation.

Divergence insufficiency: An esodeviation greater for distance vision than for near fixation, sometimes associated with intentional surgical undercorrection of esotropia.

Ductions: Monocular rotations of the eyes. Sometimes (loosely) used for relative vergences.

Eccentric fixation: A monocular condition in which a retinal point other than the fovea is used for fixation.

Essential alternation: A freely alternating strabismus. This term is usually inappropriate since one eye is generally preferred at one fixation distance or another. See, *accidental alternation*.

Fixation: The eye is positioned to align the object of regard with the fovea.

Fixation disparity: A small deviation of the eyes during normal binocular vision acting as a trigger to maintain binocular control, if compensated, but indicating potential loss of control if decompensated.

Functional amblyopia: Reduced visual acuity without a refractive or visible abnormality of the eye.

Fusional amplitudes ('fusional reserves'): See also *relative vergences*, the preferred term for horizontal amplitudes. May be applied to vertical or cyclofusional amplitudes.

Harmonious ARC: Where correspondence exists between areas on the fixing and deviating eyes which receive the same image.

Hering's law (equal innervation): Equal nerve impulses go to the agonist and its contralateral synergist.

Hess screen: A single screen for measuring incomitancy and paresis.

Horopter: The surface in physical space upon which objects lie which stimulate corresponding retinal elements in each eye.

Incomitancy: A dissymmetry of version eye movements under associated (tropia) or dissociated (phoria) conditions. The angle of the deviation varies depending upon which eye fixes, and in which direction of gaze. May be paretic or non-paretic.

Lee's screen: A transilluminated double screen for measuring incomitancy and paresis.

Localization, absolute: The patient's position in space determined from binocular information.

Localization, relative: The position of visual objects with reference to each eye, separately.

Microtropia: Any small angle squint intermediate between heterophoria and heterotropia (see Chapter 4).

Microtropia with identity: Microtropia where the angles of the deviation, (ARC) anomaly, and of monocular eccentric fixation are identical (see 7.13).

Middle third rule: The fixation point should be within the middle third of the total positive and negative relative vergence range (see 6.9).

Monofixational phoria: A small angle deviation, intermediate between a phoria and a tropia as defined by Parks (1969). It is simpler to use the wider description of microtropia.

Myotomy: Incision into or across the belly of a muscle to weaken its action. Commonly used to describe a weakening procedure on the inferior obliques.

Near point of accommodation (NPA): The nearest point at which an object can be seen clearly.

Normal retinal correspondence (NRC): A common visual direction is shared by the two foveas and all other retinal elements of each eye share equal visual directions, based on their angular subtense from the fovea.

Normo-sensorial esotropia: A rare form of non-accommodative squint with no sensory adaptation; one eye may be closed or covered to avoid diplopia (see 7.5).

Occlusion: One eye is covered to exclude vision completely, partially or segmentally. Segmental occlusion may be applied to both eyes simultaneously, e.g. bi-nasal occlusion.

Ocular torticollis: A head tilt and/or turn adopted to minimize the effect of a vertical paresis, usually a congenital paresis.

Ophthalmoplegia: Paralysis of some or all of the extra- and/or intra-ocular muscles.

Organic amblyopia: Reduced visual acuity due to a visible abnormality of the eye.

Orthophoria: The visual axes remain aligned with the object of regard, even on extended occlusion of either eye.

Palsy: See, *paralysis, paresis.*

Panum's fusional space: An area around corresponding retinal points, including slightly disparate retinal elements, whose stimulations will result in binocular fusion with stereopsis rather than diplopia.

Paradoxic diplopia: Temporary persistence or re-appearance of pre-operative ARC resulting in diplopia. This term should not be used as once the cause is understood, it cannot be paradoxic. It should be described as unharmonious ARC.

Paralysis (palsy): Complete loss of action of a muscle.

Paresis (palsy): Partial loss of action of a muscle.

Past-pointing:
(1) In recent paresis, a motor anomaly found when an object is fixated by the paretic eye in the direction of action of the paretic muscle; it appears further from the primary position than it actually is, and will cause past-pointing.
(2) A sensory anomaly found in gross eccentric fixation. When the amblyopic eye fixates, the image falling on the eccentric point is localized (and pointed) to the opposite side to the eccentricity.

Phi phenomenon: (loosely used to describe) The object being fixated appears to jump during alternate cover testing in heterophoria, and when the fixing eye is covered in tropia due to image movement across the retina.

Physiological diplopia: Where an object is situated closer or beyond the horopter and its extension forming Panum's fusional space, its image will fall on non-corresponding retinal points of each eye and so will be seen double during normal binocular vision.

Pleoptics: The diagnosis and treatment of neglected or severe functional amblyopia, often with eccentric fixation, using light stimulation and related methods.

Primary deviation (angle): The angle of deviation when the non-paretic eye is fixing.

Primary position: The direction of gaze when both eyes fixate an object at infinity, on the midline, without elevation or depression of the eyes.

Prism vergence: See, *relative vergence*.

Recession: The insertion of a muscle is dissected and re-attached (medial rectus: from 3−6 mm) posteriorly, so weakening its action.

Redress, movement of: An extra back and forth horizontal movement after an eye has made a re-fixation movement in the alternate cover test. The angle is assessed as being neutralized when the extra movement in each direction is equal.

Relative fusional convergence: Converging with fixed accommodation.

Relative fusional divergence: Divergence with fixed accommodation.

Relative vergences (amplitudes, fusional reserves): The horizontal motor range over which normal sensory perception (binocular single vision) can be maintained. A positive relative vergence relates to adduction, negative to abduction.

Resection: Shortening a muscle (lateral rectus: from 5−15 mm) and re-attaching it at the original insertion, thus strengthening its action.

Retinal element: Any small area on the retina.

Retinal rivalry: Alternating suppression and simultaneous perception of all or part of both visual fields. Typically occurs when dissimilar images fall on corresponding areas, especially with a decompensated phoria, e.g. with a fixation disparity test.

Secondary deviation (angle): The (larger) angle of deviation paresis when the paretic eye is fixing.

Sherrington's law (reciprocal innervation): Equal innervation to contract and to relax is sent to the agonist and the ipsilateral antagonist respectively.

Single mirror haploscope: An adjustable stereoscope utilizing real space, with a working distance of 1 m. It is used for the measurement and treatment of phorias and tropias.

Synergist: A muscle utilizing its primary or secondary action to assist the agonist.

Synoptophore: A stereoscope whose monocular targets may be independently aligned to measure and treat any deviation.

Tenectomy: Partial or complete excision of a muscle tendon.

Tenotomy: Partial or complete excision of a muscle.

Torsion: A rotatory movement of an eye about its anterior–posterior axis. Where a different amount of torsion occurs between the two eyes, cyclophoria or cyclotropia exists.

Unharmonious ARC: Where correspondence appears to exist between retinal areas on the fixing and deviating eyes which do not receive the same image. Unless the patient complains of diplopia, unharmonious ARC is an artefact of the testing equipment.

Vergences: Disjugate eye movements.

Versions: Conjugate eye movements.

Visual axis: The projection from the fovea through the nodal point of the eye.

Visual direction (local sign): The property of the cortical representation of a retinal element, to project images received on the retinal element to a specific point in space. The point in space will always be at the same angular subtense to the fovea.

Index